THE TREE OF LIFE

THE TREE OF LIFE

THE ANTI-CANCER DIET

Chris Woollams M.A. (Oxon)

Second Edition: June 2004

A catalogue record for this book is available from the British Library.

First published in June 2003 by:
Health Issues Ltd
The Elms, Radclive Road, Gawcott, Buckingham, MK18 4JB
Tel: 01280 815166
Fax: 01280 824655
E-mail: enquiries@iconmag.co.uk

Second Edition published June 2004

Cover design by Jeremy Baker.

ISBN 0-9542968-4-2

Printed in Great Britain by Bath Press Ltd, Lower Bristol Road, Bath, BA2 3BL

"Research is for the guidance of wise men, and the obedience of fools".

(David Ogilvy)

Important Notice

This book represents a review and an interpretation of a vast number of varied sources available to anyone on the subject of diet, healthy eating, and cancer, its prevention and possible cure.

Whilst the author has made every effort to ensure that the facts, information and conclusions are accurate and as up-to-date as possible at the time of publication, the author and publisher assume no responsibility.

The author is neither a fully qualified health practitioner nor a doctor of medicine and so is not qualified to give any advice on any medical matters. Cancer (and its related illnesses) is a very serious and very individual disease, and readers must consult with experts and specialists in the appropriate medical field before taking, or refraining from taking, any action.

This book and the advice contained are not intended as an alternative to such specialist advice, which should be sought for accurate diagnosis and before any course of treatment.

The author and the publisher cannot be held responsible for any action, or lack of action, that is taken by any reader as a result of information contained in the text of this book. Such action is taken entirely at the reader's own risk.

For all people who like their food, yet want to beat cancer, the biggest threat to life in the Western World.

CONTENTS

SECTION C – THE 'ANTI-CANCER' DIET

PREFACE

Can one book really change your life forever?

As some of you may know, in the last year I have given speeches on cancer in the UK, America and Australia. After these, many people came up to me and ask what they should be eating to best help them beat their cancer, or to prevent cancer in the first place.

The World Health Organisation has, after all, confirmed that in their view 70 per cent of cancers are caused by poor diet and 40 per cent of all cancers could be prevented by simple changes in diet. (How they marry those two figures is their business!)

It is anyway a little too rigid to think of 70 per cent of cancers being caused by one thing, and 10 per cent by another.

Although toxic products like asbestos can cut through the whole cancer process, I prefer to think of life as a tall building, the foundations of which are based on diet. Get the foundations wrong and it weakens the whole structure allowing other factors to come along and cause the weakened building to finally collapse.

But where does healthy eating to prevent cancer end and the requirements for a healthy diet start? The lines actually blur. At the moment we are introducing plans for cancer prevention in school curricula in the North East of England. The idea of protective and healthy foods is actually important in the prevention of all diseases, not just cancer. However the stark facts are that one in two men and one in three women alive today will get cancer.

Cancer is a multi-stage, complex disease of the fundamental metabolism of the body.

Cancer is systemic. Although it happens to appear in one place first, its effects exist throughout the body. Unless you attend to the fundamental causes of cancer, no localised treatment like surgery or radiotherapy can hope to succeed in the long term and it is quite likely that your cancer may reappear again, even possibly in another part of your body. It is also important to realise that unless you build your own personal and healthy microclimate in a world that is trying to pollute you, you will most likely fall victim to a cancer at some point in your lives.

Realise now that beating cancer is in your own hands as much, if not more, than it lies with any doctor. Professor Karol Sikora, formerly of the WHO, and now at Hammersmith Hospital has said exactly this in public frequently.

Of course, it's not just the food in your diet you have to attend to. I could write a whole book on toxins in the environment you need to avoid – but that is for another day. However there are several aspects of your broader 'diet' you need to start with including:

- Your water and its cleanliness,
- The air, and the oxygen in your blood,
- The exercise you take, and its effect on your metabolism,
- Your ability to control your weight and to be as proud of your body as you are of your home, your car or your achievements.

The more people talked to me, the more the cliché list of food and diet claims expanded, and the more confused people seemed to be. "*Vegetarian is best*"; "*the newspaper said to eat high carbohydrate and low fat*"; "*why do the French eat so much fat and get away with it?*"; "*I know the Japanese have less cancer, but soya disagrees with me"; "Why is it all diets just tell me what I can't eat?*". And so on.

Hardly a week seems to go by without another 'diet' hitting the papers, although most are concerned with losing weight, which is not necessarily the same as being healthy. And when it comes to healthy eating there are many pitfalls. There are individuals' views based on personal experiences; there are views that emanate covertly from the marketing departments of food companies or agricultural bodies, and there are even the often limited views of Western governments and some leading charities. Many are biased, many out-of-date, many superficial and many do not take account of modern knowledge in nutrition or biochemistry. For example there have been several important research studies in recent years on the effect of vitamins K and D with cancer, yet in both cases government Recommended Daily

Allowances (RDAs) for supplements are based on 60-year-old data for non-cancer diseases like rickets.

So I decided to start again; to go through all the research, from Nobel prize winning papers to Japanese studies on rural mushroom growers. I read the books, talked to some of the world's top nutritionists and to the doctors and nurses involved in cancer clinics.

I also remembered that when Catherine, my 22-year-old daughter, developed her cancer we didn't really stop her eating things so much as we added foods *into* her diet. Foods like garlic and isoflavones which can stop essential blood vessels that the tumour needs to form, or foods like pumpkin seeds and sunflower seeds for key antioxidant vitamins and minerals, or lentils for protective phytoestrogens.

And this led me to ***The Tree of Life***. I used the symbol of a tree so you can see easily what underpins the 'diet', what supports it and that the volume of the total diet should be in the highly protective branches, and the foliage and fruit of the tree. *The Tree of Life* is a healthy eating programme that is based on real scientific evidence and tells you what foods you need to **add** into your diets, not simply take out. It's a plan that helps your body get back into balance with the environment as much as possible, despite the toxins being thrown at you. And most of all it's an **easy** diet. Easy to understand, easy to use. Whether you have cancer or just want to prevent it.

The Tree of Life is a healthy eating plan; a programme of additions not omissions and this book simply aims to convey everything you need to know to help you in your desire to eat well yet, for example, beat cancer. Probably the most obvious discovery in preparing this book was that we have simply just stopped eating the foods that best protect us.

I would like to add one, albeit slightly controversial, point.

Orthodox medicine has three main weapons in the fight against cancer: surgery, radiotherapy and chemotherapy. It is not my intention to argue that diet should replace any of these, although clearly if the World Heath Organisation have concluded poor diet can cause a cancer, logic dictates that a good diet could well correct it.

Sadly, some medical authorities and some doctors seem to fear this possibility and, whilst paying lip service to a mantra of, 'eat five lots of fruit and vegetables a day,' do much in their power to ridicule or belittle cancer patients' dietary and supplement taking efforts. At the offices of **icon**, our magazine, we know. We have several phone calls each week from cancer patients who have been told their dietary efforts are worthless, their supplements unnecessary. This is both upsetting and worrying for them. It is also completely inaccurate and positively mischievous. Why do some doctors and scientists take this misleading and unnecessary position? Only they know. To these few people I offer the words of George Bernard Shaw: *"It is easy . . . terribly easy . . . to shake a man's faith in himself. To take advantage of that, to break a man's spirit, is the devil's work."*

Diet is an essential weapon in the fight against cancer. Use that weapon.

Finally I should like to thank my daughter, Catherine, for preparing such excellent recipes, my friend Larry Brooks for kick-starting the project, and Lindsey Fealey, for yet again putting up with the hard work and, at times, downright panic in making deadlines.

Thanks also to Dr Rob Verkerk for helping me with the water chapter, Gerald Green for his expertise on yeasts and Lawrence Plaskett, Dr Contreras and Charlotte Gerson for spending so much time with me.

SECTION A

SEEKING KNOWLEDGE

PART I

FIRST PRINCIPLES

CHAPTER 1
A DIET OF MISINFORMATION

"*An apple a day keeps the doctor away. Especially if well aimed*".

Mark Twain obviously had his own theories on diet. Indeed the common apple contains large quantities of potassium but little sodium, good quantities of magnesium, cancer protecting flavenoids, quercitin, polypeptides, glycoproteins and the ability to help you have an alkaline cellular environment. Its pips contain B-17 whilst the whole apple contains helpful vitamins and fibre. So all in all it is highly protective, healthy and anti-carcinogenic. Not bad for a projectile missile, Mark!

I've been studying cancer, in enormous depth, for four years, since my daughter Catherine became ill with the disease. However, before that I'd spent six years studying nutrition and body energy systems and, some thirty-something years ago, I read biochemistry and even spent time studying cancer research at Oxford.

In these last few very intensive years I've made a lot of friends and contacts around the world, from all fields of orthodox, complementary and alternative medicine. I've been introduced to the latest research but, when it comes to a 'healthy diet', I'm amazed how superficial most of the conclusions in many of the so-called 'healthy eating' or 'diet' books are. All too often they deteriorate into a collection of ethnic recipes.

Of course 'diet' is, in itself, a terribly ambiguous word. To the great majority of women, say the word diet and they will answer, "which one?", or "oh, no!" Diet to them is a wearing experience, synonymous with cutting certain, often enjoyable, foods out of their normal daily lives.

Nowhere more so than so-called 'healthy eating' diets like, the 'vegetarian diet' or the 'South East Asian diet', where participants seem to give up more than they actually consume!

No wonder Dr Gerson in the USA and Dr Plaskett in the UK refer to their 'diets' as Therapies. The basic principle of The Gerson Therapy, updated in line with modern findings in biochemistry and nutrition by Dr Lawrence Plaskett in the UK, was that the illness of cancer resulted from a fundamental 'poisoning' of the body's cellular metabolism. Clear out the 'poisoning' and the body's metabolic processes should start functioning properly again, and with that the full ability of the immune system to kick out the cancer. The organic vegetable and fruit diet, plus hourly juices, added supplements and coffee enemas worked for Oxford don, Michael Gearin-Tosh as chronicled in his book *Living Proof: A Medical Mutiny*, just as it has worked for many others with a variety of diseases over the past fifty years. Charlotte Gerson is a testimony to the preventive powers of the diet herself. To meet her is to find a healthy vibrant 55-year-old (she is in fact 80!). However, some people find the Therapy with its five coffee enemas per day a little extreme.

Is meat eating wrong?

Furthermore, to study a single culture and present their 'diet' as the Holy Grail can be misleading. For example, the Oxford Study on vegetarians and their diets concluded that they had 40 per cent less cancer than equivalent meat eaters. Other information has to be factored in, for example: What if I told you that vegetarians are 80 per cent less likely to smoke or drink excess alcohol? To what degree does this contribute to their 40 per cent reduced risk of cancer? Clearly diet is merely a part of their whole lifestyle and it is this which gives them 40 per cent less cancers. Maybe the diet, per se, is not so good after all!!

Please believe me I'm not trying to be facetious here. I have received a couple of letters from indignant vegetarians saying that all the evidence points to a meat-free diet being highly protective and it is true that, for example, the Bristol Cancer Help Centre recommend a vegetarian diet for people with cancer.

To me this all seems too simplistic. Yes, we know that animal fat brings with it dissolved toxins from the fields plus the animal's hormones, but would lean free-range game be so wrong? And just as the Okinawans, who eat wild meat and fish, live longer than vegetarians, so too do a number of other populations. Sally Beare in her recent book *The Live Longer Diet* has studied longevity in various populations.

Moreover, one man's meat is really and truly another's poison. Peter D'Adamo has written a very good book on choosing the right foods for your blood type: *Eat Right for Your Type*. In this he tracks how populations moved out of Africa and developed different blood types around the world. These different types actually thrive on different foods, for example one type thriving on meat eating whilst another thrives on vegetarianism.

Some treatment clinics have developed this theory with good results. Indeed, none of this is new. It dates back to a Scottish scientist called John Beard who in 1906 developed views on how cancer cells formed. Although his work disappeared in the 1930s as trendy new therapies like radiotherapy and then chemotherapy emerged, it reemerged in the USA with a dentist called William Kelley.

Kelley developed quite an intricate version of metabolic typing. Perhaps the most significant event during his studies was that his wife developed cancer and he successfully treated her with a vegetarian diet. Yet when he, himself, developed cancer a vegetarian diet had absolutely no effect. However, a significant improvement occurred when he started eating meat three times a day!

In the end, he developed twelve metabolic sub-types (see *Everything You Need to Know to Help You Beat Cancer*), and his work is now continued at the highly successful Gonzalez clinic in New York. Bill Wolcott, who worked with Kelley, has developed a whole system of metabolic typing to show you which foods your personal biochemistry is best suited to. These may be vegetarian-based or they may include meat and fish (www.healthexcel.com).

The so-called 'South East Asian diet' is very similar to a vegetarian diet; Western observers most notably cite its predominance of vegetables, rice and soya. With Chinese breast cancer rates in the 2–6 per 100,000 women range and a figure of 38 per 100,000 in Scotland, it is 'in vogue' to talk about the diet's health and anti-cancer benefits and a hundred recipe books have been spawned. But how many Chinese women take the pill or HRT? How many use hair colourings, perfumes or cosmetics with their oestrogen mimicking ingredients, all found to play a role in increased rates of the disease called cancer?

Let's try another line of thought.

What if I told you that vegetarians also had 60 per cent less obesity than meat eaters and that being overweight had a direct link to a variety of illnesses from diabetes to cancer? (For example, the Fred Hutchinson Center in Seattle has linked obesity in women with 20 per cent more breast cancers.)

Or that the Bush people, like South East Asians do eat meat and yet they all have longer life expectancies than Western vegetarians, once child mortality is removed from the statistics?

Or that the Okinawans, who eat fish and a little meat, and coral mineral-enhanced fruit and vegetables, but consume 40 per cent less calories than even the Japanese, have the highest life expectancy of them all? Both groups of people have reducing blood pressure as they age, unlike Western vegetarians and the majority of the Western world. Maybe the issue is not meat at all, but calories consumed, salt levels, or specific protective elements in the food?

Government advice?

For 20 years in the Western world we have been told by our governments to eat a high carbohydrate, low fat diet. But, in the light of modern nutrition and biochemical studies is this actually correct?

High carbohydrate diets, in the sedentary Western world, usually result in an excess of calories consumed over daily needs. This excess gets stored . . . as fat. And fat is a wonderful solvent; dissolving and holding toxins and hormones inside the body that should otherwise be excreted. Excess toxins and hormones that are more likely to cause cancer. Worse, the great majority of carbohydrate consumed in the West is 'refined', yet the FSA in the UK tells us to build a balanced diet around 'starchy foods'. This advice can lead to high insulin, diabetes, shorter lives and even cancer!

The peoples of the Bush, Okinawa and South East Asia have proven to us that current advice is wrong. They have limited calorie, **whole** grain diets. Even studies with rats show that calorie deprivation results in increased longevity. The Norwegians had their food supplies dramatically reduced by the occupying Germans during the Second World War, yet their restricted diets of fish and lowered calories resulted in a 35 per cent overall health improvement.

When people from South East Asia come to the West their cancer risk adjusts in line with Western risk levels because they are no longer 'deprived' in what they eat. They consume, and consume. And they have more illness. In the USA 26 per cent of the population are obese, and it is getting worse. Looking at their 16-year-old children, 60 per cent are overweight or obese! The data shows that being overweight increases your risk of any cancer by at least 40 per cent. Even smoking increases it by 'only' 25 per cent.

Let's try another line of thought.

Where is the evidence that proves eating a low fat diet is correct advice?

The French eat more fat than the British or the Americans and have lower heart attack rates and lower cancer rates. In fact, in Gascony, the home of foie gras, the levels of fat consumption are the highest in France, and where do you think the risk of heart attack and cancer is at its lowest? Gascony!

Eskimos consume more fat than almost any other population in the world. And historically, which group of people had virtually no cancer? The Eskimos.

The problem is that too many commentators do not look into **all** the research. They pick out the bits that suit their arguments. And as a result myths are created and perpetuated.

Nowadays almost anybody can say that the peoples of South East Asia get less cancer so why not copy their diets? And then they turn out a recipe book. After all, Thai food is the new Chinese and it is so much more interesting than standard Western fare! But cancer is not a fashion fad.

The people who do this have rarely balanced all the research, and hardly ever have they gone beneath the findings to find the links and the common themes. Research such as this is not for the obedience of wise men.

In fact, just as there are items you might cut out of your diet, like sugar, salt and nutritionally empty calorie stores like the ubiquitous refined pasta, there are things you should add in, like pulses, garlic, fish oils, nuts, olive oil and ginger, **all of which are highly protective**.

Moreover, why should we obediently copy these 'foreign' diets anyway? Where is the logic in this? It confounds the theories of metabolic typing and most definitely of evolution. Anybody who has really studied the principles of macrobiotics or naturopathy would understand that each of us, two hundred or more years ago had evolved to be in perfect balance with our **localised** environment. This balance occurs over hundreds of thousands of years and hundreds of generations. 'Recent' additions like wheat or dairy can 'throw out' this balance, as can pesticides, diesel fumes and HRT pills. But so too might importing a previously unused foodstuff like soya from 12,000 miles away even though it is helpful the other side of the globe.

Clearly the peoples of South East Asia have merely had their environments and their balance less disturbed than we have in the West. In rural China, when I was there, it was easy to imagine that many aspects of their lives had hardly changed in the last thousand years. In Thailand, a country with the same population as the UK yet only 60,000 cases of cancer per year (UK cancer level: 270,000), the Health Minister was on the front page of the Bangkok newspaper telling Thais to go back to their traditional rice, vegetable and fruit diets and to keep clear of 'dangerous' Western foods. He then cited McDonalds, KFC, Starbucks and Pizza Hut! In Europe or America, he would have been sued!

In South East Asia they have **their** balance. In England 300 years ago we had **ours**. We have just forgotten it; that's the real truth!

South East Asians eat lots of vegetables, fruit and a little soya, all of which provide phytoestrogens which can be protective in combating the effects of human oestrogens within the body.

Three hundred years ago in Europe, we consumed a lot of phytoestrogens too. Not just from vegetables but pulses, like peas, beans, lentils and flageolets. In 1900, 30 per cent of our protein consumption in the UK was plant protein from pulses. Now it is just 2 per cent. And with it has gone the protection of these pulses' phytoestrogens. Now, 47 per cent of children in the UK do not eat a vegetable other than a potato in an average week! And they receive no protection against the increasing toxins in their lives, most of which reduce the effectiveness of their immune systems. A recent survey of UK eating habits showed that children who did not eat fruit went on **almost inevitably** to get cancer later in their lives.

Why do we want to adopt the diet of another corner of the world? Why do we want to import 'magical' ingredients like soya when we have our perfectly acceptable phytoestrogen equivalents here? Ones that used to keep us balanced with our own environment. Who says taking a few of 'their' elements of balance can fully integrate us with 'our' different micro-environment?

Is it really any surprise that soya consumption is met with intolerances? At most we have only been consuming it since the 1960s in the Western world! Charlotte Gerson, quite correctly, says that soya causes allergies and also contains phytic acid and this prevents full absorption of minerals. But the Gerson Therapy decrees that the patient should maximise their vitamin and mineral intake so it advises against it. Similarly, almost all beans and pulses contain phytic acid and it advises against those too. But we have consumed peas, broad beans, lentils and chickpeas in Europe for thousands of years without allergies. Maybe the problem just lies in our Western body's relationship with this new fangled soya? I am a great fan of soya, but for Westerners only in moderation.

When did you last shell some peas or broad beans – our national phytoestrogens? As you can probably tell, already, I have little time for the current trend, or fad, where partially informed people cite the health of 'populations in South East Asia' and immediately write diets for people living in Britain based around chillies, soya and pak-choi.

Research is for the guidance of wise men and the obedience of fools. I have no intention of being foolish, and nor should you.

Finally, what of the role of doctors and health authorities in all this? I am totally supportive of all doctors, nurses and their many helpers. They deserve our praise. Anybody who spends up to seven years learning and passing exams and then dedicates their lives to saving others, fully deserves our respect.

But I wouldn't ask them about my diet, my vitamins, my nutrition, my biochemistry or my body energy levels. They are rarely qualified to give me any advice on these subjects. They have most likely never fully studied them, so how would they know? Of course patients do ask them and they do give advice like, "*eat five lots of fruit and vegetables a day*" or "*you don't need supplements if you are eating a balanced diet*". Where is the hard scientific evidence in our modern world for these two well-worn answers?

Sadly, many people listen to this rubbish. It is not the fault of the doctors themselves, of course. The exams they are set and the training they receive, means that they could qualify without spending one day learning about nutrition, biochemistry or body energy, three fundamental pillars of good health.

It is clearly time that the health authorities woke up to modern knowledge levels and discoveries. Instead we see 'sensational' headlines in the press, for example "*vitamins are useless – even for cancer*", stemming from a study that was nothing to do with cancer and was actually designed to look at cholesterol blockers called statins on heart attack rates amongst people who have already been diagnosed as **heart** patients. Such sensationalism is nonsense, and dangerously misleading to a population who already feel confused by the inconsistencies coming from the medical authorities.

Only recently a number of scientists published a paper in the *British Journal of Cancer* 2004 90, 408–13. These scientists (Wernecke, Earl, Seydel, Horn, Crichton and Fannon) are associated with major UK hospitals. The report started with the statement, "Many cancer patients use complementary alternative medicines (CAMs) but may not be aware of the potential risks. There are no studies quantifying such risks, but there is some evidence of patient risk from case reports in the literature". This was in fact a complete *non sequitur* from the focus of the report. Namely a simple study of patients (318 took part) to find out who was taking what. 60.4 per cent were female, and 51.6 per cent took herbal remedies and/or food supplements. There were a few more results about types of supplement taken, but that basically was the research study.

However the report actually went on for about six pages listing various warnings for everything from cod liver oil to echinacea. In the body copy it quoted studies and tests 'against' certain vitamins, but never any 'for', when in fact there are hundreds, maybe thousands. Indeed, as you will see in Chapter 18, John Boik of the prestigious MD Anderson Cancer Institute in Texas completed a book in March 2001 called *Natural Compounds in Cancer Therapy*, listing over 4000 references.

These six scientists also included within the article the statement "our survey highlights the importance for conventional healthcare professionals to discuss CAM use with their patients". But which doctor or oncologist is fully aware of the numerous detailed studies on vitamin E with cancer, or that there are twenty positive studies on beta-carotene?

Subjective choices on pieces of research, in a paper actually about a research study on another, albeit associated, topic do little to reassure the public that the medical authorities have their best interests at heart. Within days, of course, news media have picked up that 'CAMs' are dangerous. This is really most misleading and unhelpful.

There has been so much advancement in our knowledge of nutrition and cellular biochemistry over the last twenty years that all the authorities have to do is be able to read and absorb. Oh, and have an open mind. For every vitamin, we have reported in **icon** probably ten good studies on its benefits with cancer. They are right to criticise the 'faddism' of many alternative approaches, but wrong not to objectively analyse the latest scientific research fully themselves, to train doctors in the knowledge, nor make serious efforts in the areas of prevention and healthy eating advice to the nation. If one takes the budget of 'screening' out of the prevention equation, for every hundred pounds spent on cancer in Britain, less than 20 pence is spent on genuine prevention and education.

As a result, even Nobel Prize winners are ignored. The work of Sir John Vane on the development of a negative and toxic environment for our cells and how to avoid it, happened in the late 1970s. In 2000 the Mayo Clinic was repeating part of the work and coming up with the same findings. When I rang the major charity helplines about why they were not passing on the message that studies have now proven and re-proven the benefits of omega 3 (fish oils) and aspirin (try aloe vera instead) in combating cancer, they simply said they had no knowledge of either piece of research. In 2002 alone I counted more than six major pieces of international research yet again confirming the 'omega 3 and/or aspirin help beat cancer' theory – by April 2003 it was American research saying aspirin beats breast cancer. Why do we waste so much money reinventing the wheel? Why can't we just read and learn?

Worse, the *BJC* article mentioned above actually quotes warnings for cod liver oil, evening primrose oil and garlic all of which "can interfere with warfarin, aspirin and non-steroidal anti-inflammatory drugs" without mentioning any of the research confirming their benefits. Frankly if it's a choice between rat poison and cod liver oil, I know which one I'll be using!

The fact is that cod liver oil, garlic, ginger, aspirin and the like all act in the same way and numerous studies have shown this (see Eicosanoids, later).

Another major achievement being ignored, Gunter Blöbel's 1998 Nobel Prize for glycoproteins shows us how cells can receive messages. Further work on this has led to the finding that certain mono- and polysaccharides are essential in our diet to 'detox' our cells and let our natural defensive killers recognise developing rogue cancer cells. However even though we are eating less and less of these polysaccharides in our foods, the new EU directives will not allow the sale of any supplements that might improve glycoprotein or polysaccharide levels in the human body. They simply are not on the approved list. One wonders if they even read the research? (Don't worry, these ingredients may be obtained from foods, if you know what to eat – see Chapter 18.)

The cynics would say that these two Nobel Prizes are ignored because the resulting helpful foods and ingredients cannot be patented and turned into expensive and profitable drugs (although that doesn't stop the pharmaceutical companies who are currently working hard on patentable derivative drugs, and will only 'shout' out the news in about 7 years or so when they have completed all the tests!). One firm in the USA has already picked up on Blöbel's work and formulated a new patented product called Arithroprotein; after just 9 months it is a $2.2 billion brand. We'll see if it gets EU approval, shall we?

In February 2004 a study was produced in the UK by David Thomas on the severe declining mineral levels in fruit and vegetables. The FSA derided the research saying the methods of analysis in 1940 and 1990 were different. When asked, they made no comment on the actual findings of huge losses of calcium, iron, magnesium and potassium merely repeating the government advice to eat five lots of fruit and vegetables a day. However, these results were confirmed by a second study (Anne-Marie Mayer of Cornell University).

"*Nothing is more terrible than ignorance in action*" (Goethe).

CHAPTER 2
ADDING FOODS INTO YOUR DIET

The aim of this book is to distil all the available research information into an easy to understand, healthy diet plan that, in particular, can help people beat cancer. Whether they have it already or not, and then to provide an easy to manage programme.

Specifically, this book will focus on those foods you can **add** into your diet to afford you greater protection, based on established research evidence and epidemiology studies. So this really is an eat to beat cancer diet!

Of course this book will warn you of foods and ingredients we think it is wiser to avoid, but by and large this diet is not a diet of omission, or a 'cut this out or else' plan. A great many people find limited and rigid diets quite depressing. And depression can have very negative effects on your health. Benjamin Franklin said, "*Wealth is not his who has it, but his who enjoys it.*" Eating is not simply refueling. Eating, like wealth, should be a pleasurable and happy experience.

This healthy eating plan is called *The Tree of Life*, because it is a positive, life-enhancing plan. The tree's roots are the basics that sustain and build a healthy life: food, water, air, exercise and weight control. The trunk, the tree's stability, suggests how to maximise your vitamins and minerals. The branches determine the expanse of the tree; for these are the foods we have found that clearly protect against cancer, which neutralise toxins and which make an overall positive contribution to your health. The foliage is the vegetables and fruits, the volume of the tree and the foods that should be the volume of your diet.

Western vegetarians may have 40 per cent less cancer risk than non-vegetarians, but research shows we can also reduce our risks of cancer by the same factor if we take omega 3 regularly, or selenium, or a host of other vitamins and supplements. Or if we eat natural foods like oily fish, nuts and garlic. So, given that 60 million people in Britain are **not** vegetarians, actually like meat and are never likely to give it up, there seems to be little point in constantly telling them about vegetarianism when more modest 'pruning' of certain food stuffs might be all that is necessary as long as they are prepared to actually add certain things into their diet. To get back to some of the things that used to keep us healthy.

Above all *The Tree of Life* is about realism.

The 'French paradox' referred to in Chapter 1, is usually ignored by most commentators as it sits uneasily with a superficial review of the information from the Far East, or vegetarian studies.

The French eat more fat than the Americans and British, and consume more wine. Yet they have lower rates of cancer and heart diseases, they spend 30 per cent less on health care and enjoy a longer average life expectancy.

These trends tend to be more acute in the areas bordering the northern Mediterranean where diets typically include:

- A limited amount of meat
- A limited amount of dairy (from cows)
- Red wine consumption with meals
- Good consumption of fresh nuts
- Good consumption of dried fruits
- High consumption of vegetables, including garlic
- High consumption of whole grains
- High consumption of fruits
- High consumption of olive oils and nut oils (monounsaturated oils)
- High percentage of home-grown, in season, fresh and organic produce
- High consumption of fish.

We will analyse the specific benefits of this diet later in the book, but suffice it to say it is packed with foods that are naturally protective, like fish oils and omega 3, olive oil, nut oils, garlic, red peppers, tomatoes, green vegetables, and (oh, yes) red wine. The list is endless. Indeed the principles behind it of local, in season vegetables and fruit, and high whole grain content are very similar to those defined by the Japanese originator of the macrobiotic diet. And the diet has a huge number of elements in common with South East Asian diets, so already common themes of importance are being found.

Why should the same principles not apply to the basic British or Americans diet? Why can we not remember what foods used to protect us within our natural environments? Why have we thrown them all away, and with them our natural health too?

Why do we neglect our own apples, yet import apples from other countries? Or demand exotic fruits, often picked unripe (when the vitamin content has not fully formed), and transport them for days (by which time much of the remaining vitamins have gone) to then 'ripen' them up in a shop window locally? We are in fact eating unripe, rotting, vitamin-deficient pineapples and bananas, when we could be eating our own pears!

The Tree of Life is not a diet of omission; it is a scientifically based approach to adding natural health protectors into your lives in the state that makes them most effective. Living foods for healthy living.

What we have looked for is commonalities. We are more interested in principles than actual foods. The Mediterranean peoples may have their antioxidant drink, but so too do the Asians. One man's honey is another's red wine, or another's green tea. What types of foods protect the peoples of South East Asia, that also protect the peoples of the Mediterranean, or the Kalahari, or vegetarians?

Not surprisingly there are categories of food that come up in all these diets. For example, isoflavones in the pulses of France and the soya of Japan; glycoproteins in the mushrooms of Japan or the apples of England.

Then there are specific beneficial products like garlic, in the French or Chinese diets, or unadulterated sunflower oil used for cooking in Greece or Thailand. Common foods underpinning healthy benefits.

We have foods that have kept us healthy wherever we live, for thousands of years. Maybe we just need to remind ourselves of them.

CHAPTER 3

ATOMIC MAN – PERFECT BALANCE

At least 95 per cent of you and I is air although, to look at each of us, it is hard to imagine. Because every molecule in your body is made of atoms and these are simply electrons spinning around neutrons. Both electrons and neutrons are infinitesimally small particles, and between them, relatively speaking, are huge spaces or air masses.

Atoms attract and repel other atoms; atoms help other atoms do their job; atoms control how your cell's systems work and how well they work; the right atoms control your health and well-being, or your lack of it and illness.

Your atoms and their electronic fields are affected by all manner of external atoms and their electronic fields. The influence of radiation from a mobile phone, power cables, microwaves and x-rays is easiest to understand.

More than this, every day you exchange millions of atoms with your environment, every time you breathe, or eat or drink. So much so that every 90 days the great majority of the body's tissues have atoms that are completely new to the body.

The presence of too many of one atom might completely overwhelm the presence of another; too many of one atom might prevent another from doing its job, inhibit its action or stop it working altogether.

It is easy to see how you might poison your metabolism quite quickly. But it is also easy to see how your recovery is equally possible.

The fully healthy body works in a state of balance and harmony. It follows therefore that the unhealthy body is in a state of imbalance and disharmony.

To stand any chance of beating cancer, and of being healthy, your mental focus should be 'atomic man, in perfect balance.'

The sodium-potassium imbalance

My father used to get cramp in the night, so the doctor told him to eat more salt. This is wrong. Cramping of the muscles is caused by excess production of lactic acid. This takes place in the mitochondria, or 'power stations', inside every cell in the muscle tissue. It is caused because the power stations have run out of oxygen and are forced to burn the fuel without it. This action is very similar to the action of a cancer cell which has no choice but to burn fuel in the absence of oxygen. This action is worsened by a lack of **potassium**. Indeed excess sodium prevents potassium getting into the cell to help correct the problem!

Salt is a generic term for things that contain sodium. We ingest sodium as salt or sea salt (sodium chloride); or preservative salt in meats and other foods (sodium nitrate, sodium nitrite); or taste enhancing salt (like monosodium glutamate); or in baking powder salt.

Whichever way we take our sodium, the average individual in the West consumes much, much more than they need; much, much more than makes them healthy. As animals in the wild, hundreds of thousands of years ago we ate virtually no salt. Indeed, we had to go to a salt 'lick' just to get some. By the Middles Ages salt was still a rarity and had become a currency to barter with. Hence the origins of the word salary from the Latin salarium. Salt had its place, but largely as a preservative for food stored for the winter months. From all this I could easily construct an argument that the maximum sodium intake should be around one gram per day. Yet the Food Standards Agency (FSA) says six for adults and three for children, but no detailed rationale is given. Eight grams is a more usual Western consumption, whilst the average New Yorker consumes about eight kilogrammes per year or over twenty grams per day! And that is an average figure!

In February 2004 the US Institute of Medicine published a report stating that healthy 19–50-year-olds should consume 1.25 grams of sodium per day, much nearer to the figure I have suggested. Even allowing for the weight of the chloride or nitrite, this would yield an upper 'salt' limit of around 5 grams maximum. They note that 95 per cent of American males and 75 per cent of American females exceed this figure.

In February 2004 **icon** reported on new Japanese research that showed people who ate 12–15 grams of 'salt' doubled their risk of stomach cancer (*British Journal of Cancer*, February.).

Excess sodium has a devastating effect on all cellular membranes and inhibits the correct flow of essential elements into the cell. To that end it affects everything from your brain cells, to your immune cells, and virtually all the normal and healthy metabolic processes in every cell of your body.

It is impossible to talk about sodium without talking about potassium – they are partners. Potassium is essential to the healthy workings inside your cells. Without it the cell becomes imbalanced and unhealthy. The easiest way to think of this is that sodium should largely work outside the cell, while potassium works inside the cell. Too much sodium stops potassium getting in and, worse, actually causes the kidneys to expel it from the body. If excess sodium gets inside the cell, it will prevent the proper action of potassium inside the cells and will result in serious harm. Excess sodium poisons cells. Over thousands of years, our power stations, or mitochondria, have evolved to use potassium. This is what makes them run smoothly, and potassium hydroxide is alkaline. If sodium displaces the potassium, the chemical reactions falter, the cell works inefficiently, it becomes more acid and displaces oxygen. It is on its way to being a typical oxygen-free cancer cell.

For healthy cells your intake of these two atoms should significantly favour potassium, about five to one over sodium.

Prime sources of **stressful sodium** are (approximately in milligrams):

Salt (1 teaspoon)	2000
Cheese, processed (100 gms)	1200
Cheese spread (100 gms)	1100
Oxo cube (1)	1030
Bacon (1 rasher)	1000
Chicken nuggets (6)	1000
Corned beef (100 gms)	1000
Soy sauce (1 tablespoon)	1000
Gravy and sauces (100 gms)	1000
Cornflakes (100 gms)	1000
White bread (4 slices)	900
Baking soda (1 teaspoon)	820
French fries, salted (1 portion)	750

Cheddar cheese (100 gms)	600
Sausage (1 medium)	500
MSG (1 teaspoon)	500
Baked beans, canned (100 gms)	500
Pie casing (1)	500
Cottage cheese (100 gms)	450
Soup, canned	450
Fish, canned	450
Peanuts (100 gms)	420
Fish fingers (100 gms)	400
Spaghetti hoops, canned (100 gms)	400
Biscuits (100 gms)	375
Baking powder (1 teaspoon)	350
Crisps (2 packets)	350
Butter or margarine, salted (2 tablespoons)	250

So you can see stressful sodium is found in certain categories of foods: preserved meats and sausages, condiments (from tomato ketchup to soy sauce), canned foods, breakfast cereals, bread (white or wholemeal), biscuits and cakes, all baked flour products, fast food, crisps and peanuts.

Obviously fish, particularly shellfish, contain sodium (but nowhere near the levels of bread or fast foods) and even beer and fizzy soft drinks contain quite high levels of sodium to enhance the taste!

An excess of sodium is debilitating. Apart from its potential disruptive and even cancer inducing effects inside the cell, it affects the water balance of the body and causes stress, fatigue and even depression.

Perky potassium is highly corrective of this. Potassium controls the energy production in our cellular power stations, the mitochondria, and crucially our protein and DNA synthesis. It helps in brain function, nerve transmission and muscle tone and is anti-ageing, whilst excess sodium ages tissues. If cells are depleted of potassium, pathological change occurs with damaging metabolic acids being produced and the cell is on its way to disease and even death. Furthermore a lack of potassium inside a cell, causes sodium to fill in the vacuum and sodium actually increases the metabolic acidity further causing degenerative disease and cell death. A real double-whammy.

Perky potassium can be found (approximately in milligrams) in:

Lentils (100 gms)	1400
Potato, baked with skin (medium)	1250
Broad beans and peas (100 gms)	1200
Muesli, homemade (100gms)	1000
Potatoes (250 gms)	800
Nuts (100 gms)	700
Banana (medium)	450
Fish, fresh (100 gms)	450 *
Vegetables, green leaf (100 gms)	350
Meat, lean organic (100 gms)	350
Orange (medium)	300
Rice, brown (100 gms)	250
Carrots (100 gms)	250
Apple (medium)	200

* Depends on the fish – can vary from 150–450

In all of the above, sodium levels are negligible (even in fish where it is approximately 100 mgs per 100 gms). Potassium is found in vegetables and fruit, nuts and fish, brown rice and lean organic meat (beware non-organic red meat often has sodium salts added to it to give it better colour). Parsley and garlic, those two French staples, are also good sources.

A simple rule is also that fresh food is low in sodium and high in potassium, whilst preserved, refined and prepared foods are the opposite.

The calcium–magnesium imbalance

One of the biggest and worst hoaxes portrayed to the Western world over the last fifty years is that we are deficient in calcium so we must drink more milk. If you read this in your magazine, cancel your subscription; if your doctor tells you this, change doctors!

Osteoporosis is caused, not simply by low calcium, but by low magnesium and poor vitamin D levels. (Oh, and toxins like steroids, and excesses of caffeine and sodium!)

Calcium and magnesium are partners.

Dodgy dairy inhibits the body's uptake of zinc (crucial in helping vitamin C with its cellular and anti-cancer activities), iron (crucial for maintaining the correct oxygen levels in blood and cells) and magnesium.

Without **magnificent magnesium** you cannot absorb calcium into your cellular tissues or bones. The Western world which floods its bodies with dairy, also has the lowest levels of calcium in its tissues. Recent USA research claims that 40 per cent of us are magnesium deficient.

The daily calcium requirement is just less than one gram. Amounts in excess of this will actually cause magnesium depletion and further prevent calcium absorption. Furthermore, magnesium is needed for vitamin D synthesis in the body. Low magnesium means low vitamin D levels. Low vitamin D levels mean low calcium absorption and, worse, vitamin D deficiency is linked to certain cancers from colon to brain tumours. Vitamin D supplementation is now being given as part of cancer therapies at the Royal Marsden Hospital in the UK.

Traditional healthy diets, from China to the Kalahari, or Greece to the Eskimos incorporate **no** cow's milk. Rather, they are magnesium rich. Magnificent magnesium rich.

Best foods for magnesium are nuts, pulses, melons, mango, fresh sweetcorn, jacket potato, bananas, green leaves, whole grains like millet, oats, buckwheat or wheatgerm and brown rice.

If you cut all dairy from your diet this instant, you could still get your daily calcium requirement from 150 gms of spinach; or a few almonds, haricot vert, broccoli, leeks and an orange; or dried apricots, whole grains and wheatgerm at breakfast and dinner.

Magnificent magnesium is crucial to a healthy liver; a healthy liver is your organ of detoxification and the neutraliser of free radicals.

Magnesium is also crucial to your cells because it works a little pump. This pump actually pumps sodium out of the cells and potassium in. Without it, sodium drifts back in to poison the cells, whilst potassium drifts out.

Magnesium is also crucial in the efficient working of your power stations. It prepares the fuel for burning. Without it – for example, if you are on a slimming diet – you might have terrible cravings for food when in reality you have ingested more than enough calories. Without magnesium to prepare the food you ingested and turn it into the right sort of fuel, your cells will go hungry.

Magnesium levels are also lowered by

- refining our foods – which removes magnesium from the grain
- stress and excess physical activity – which burns up magnesium in the energetic process
- tea, coffee, alcohol – which 'wash' magnesium out of the body
- high sugar, carbohydrate and fat diets – which are nutritionally empty yet require magnesium for energy production.

It is not recommended that you supplement long term with magnesium. And calcium supplements that are neither organic, nor combined with magnesium can cause more harm than good.

Finally high fibre foods and intestinal 'good' flora probiotics are recommended, since fibre creates a healthy and acidic environment in the intestine, which combined with the flora aids the absorption of minerals such as magnesium and potassium.

CHAPTER 4
HEALTHY LIVER – HEALTHY BODY

In the UK and America few of us pay any attention to our livers. We know we have one but we don't know too much about it. Worse, we mistreat it day in, day out.

Yet the people of China or Italy, look to their livers at the first sign of illness. A routine health check in Beijing consists of a doctor looking into your ears and eyes, and then at your tongue. The state of the tongue will tell you much about the state of your intestines and liver; the colour of your eyes will tell you the levels of toxins present.

In France and Italy the feeling of being a bit 'rundown' is normally met with a shrug and the explanation 'une crise de foie' – a crisis of the liver. A little too much alcohol perhaps; even something they ate; and occasionally a bit of an infection. The locals will avoid fat for a few days and eat more vegetables like artichokes, fruits like melon and drink water. Why, they even have bottled waters that are well suited to reviving a flagging liver! The brand Hepar in France is magnesium rich and sells itself on its benefit to your liver.

By contrast, I cannot remember the last time a doctor in the UK looked at my tongue, nor the last time someone said they were feeling 'a bit livery'. Whatever happened to Andrews Liver Salts?

But your life depends on your liver. It is the largest organ in your body and a very complex one at that. It has a great many important functions, none more so than its ability to detoxify the blood.

A healthy liver filters almost two pints of blood per minute.

A healthy liver also aids digestion and absorption; it metabolises fats and cholesterol aiding their excretion; it filters out dead cells, toxins, drugs, chemicals and all sorts of debris; it processes bacteria, viruses, fungi and parasites; and most importantly it is the cornerstone of a healthy immune system.

Fatty livers

A fatty liver affects more than 50 per cent of adult Americans.

Their carbohydrate and fat-rich diets cause a log-jam in the liver.

The modern world subjects a liver to a huge range of 'poisons' which impair its function: alcohol, pesticides, chemicals, antibiotics, drugs and external hormones like animal hormones, HRT and the contraceptive pill. Any and all of these poisons can damage the Kupffer cells, which are responsible for breaking down toxic matter, impairing the biochemical pathways and reducing the performance of the liver significantly.

When the liver is damaged by such toxins, it loses its efficiency to clear fats and toxins from the body, and so becomes 'clogged up'. If it cannot process the fats and help to fully defat the body, fats will build up in the blood stream and fatty deposits will occur all over the body causing all sorts of health problems. Worse, fat is an excellent solvent and so those fatty deposits will be toxin charged, keeping free radicals, hormones and toxins in various parts of the body and creating the environment for a cancer to form.

One of the main jobs of a healthy liver is to produce bile, about three pints per day. The bile, which is pigmented often green and yellow, along with its metabolic agents, the bile salts, works tirelessly to metabolise fats and cholesterol. The process involves vast numbers of small bile ducts running throughout the liver and collecting into one common bile duct, which passes directly into the intestine. About half way along this duct sits a balloon-like object, the gall bladder, whose contractions help force the bile, along with its waste products, into the intestine.

Gallstones

For some reason best known to only themselves, Western doctors like to remove the gallbladder when patients are suffering gallstones. In fact, gallstones are formed in the liver and there is a successful and natural, albeit extreme, remedy for removing them. The gallbladder has little or nothing to do with making gallstones!

Gallstones add to the problems of fatty livers and some 70 per cent of Americans have gallstones. Worse was the finding that 99.95 per cent of cancer patients in American hospitals had gallstones.

Gallstones block the bile ducts of the liver and prevent the free flow of the fats, cholesterol and toxins into the intestines. They can be small like grains of sand and often number between 300 and 3000.

They are formed by cholesterol collecting around clumps of bacteria or even pieces of dead parasite (rather like a pearl forms around sand particles), which is especially interesting as there is a school of thought that argues that every cancer patient is afflicted by microbe infection – bacteria, yeasts, parasites or virus.

Parasites abound and are on the increase. There has been a four-fold increase in fluke in British livestock since 1997, according to government figures. But parasites do not have to be large. Microscopic parasites, immune to chlorine can be carried in water systems and on exotic vegetables and fruit. Parasites damage the liver and produce toxins like aflatoxin B, which has been linked to cancer.

If the bile system is blocked and working inefficiently then the body's system for absorbing vitamins and minerals is impaired. The bile works alongside enzymes, helpful bacteria and acids in the intestine to break down fats, and then up to 95 per cent of the bile acids are normally reabsorbed and carried back to the liver.

The liver and cancer

Under normal healthy conditions the liver manufactures substances like anti-histamines essential to the immune system. In a fatty liver, the liver depletes the whole immune system around the body as it tries to cope with the shortfall in the liver detox systems.

Cancer cells love fat. Because they do not tolerate oxygen they cannot make their energy as normal cells do from carbohydrate and oxygen. Instead they burn glucose, fat, and protein. This 'anaerobic energy production' further pulls sodium into the cells and, as we saw, that makes the cells even more toxic so the cancer thrives. The end product of this fat burning is lactic acid, in itself high toxic. The only place lactic acid can be detoxified is in the liver and the end product is glucose, which is the perfect food for the cancer cell. In a way, a cancer cell is like a parasite, modifying the host's own metabolism so it can thrive. And this is on top of the downward spiral of 'liver clogging – fat producing – fat burning – lactic acid producing – liver clogging' that worsens the patient. This process is not helped by the action of radiotherapy or chemotherapy, both of which produce large numbers of dead cells that the liver has to deal with, and both of which flatten the immune system causing an impaired, overworked liver to stretch to the very limit of its resources.

What steps can we take?

We will take the extreme case, namely that of a cancer patient. People wishing to prevent a cancer should draw their own conclusions.

1. Ensure you do not have a parasite, or yeasts elsewhere in the body.
2. Severely limit your fat intake.
3. Boost your immune system.
4. Clean your liver – generally detoxing
– bile stimulation,
– a gallstone cleanse.

The issue of microbes, from yeasts to parasites will be dealt with in Part IV. Herbal parasite purges do exist and are usually a mixture of wormwood, slippery elm, Pau d'Arco, black walnut, clove and garlic, plus a number of immune system boosters. Interestingly Pau d'Arco was originally thought to be a 'cure' for cancer until its action as a yeast and parasite killer was discovered. Wormwood has been found to kill yeasts and parasites but also to have a direct effect on cancer cells (Professor Lai, University of Washington). Wormwood also debilitates certain enzymes, found in cancer cells, which are needed to accommodate the high iron levels existing in cancer cells.

Cutting the fat out of the diet is, of course, one of the key principles seen in the Gerson and Plaskett Therapies. By using an extreme vegetarian and no-fat diet, the cancer cells have to turn to the body's stored fat as a fuel source. As we said before, overweight people do get more cancers; and they also find them harder to beat because they have more fat stores.

The immune system has to be boosted. Antioxidants like beta-carotene, vitamin C, vitamin E, zinc and selenium are important, whilst aloe vera helps the immune system in many ways. Coenzyme Q10 and the spice, turmeric, are antioxidants which will specifically help the liver.

Diets high in saturated fats, refined carbohydrates and damaging polyunsaturated fats cause the liver to produce triglycerides. Free radicals can literally provide the spark to ignite these to become dangerous and aggressive. Vitamin E and selenium work in the liver to neutralise these. Turmeric and the B vitamins, especially choline and inositol (found in soya lecithin), will also keep these in check. Meanwhile lycopene also bonds to these fatty free radicals in the blood to neutralize them.

Boldo tea strengthens the gall bladder as does globe artichoke, both promoting the excretion of fatty bile. Beets and radishes also get the juices going, as do green salads, green vegetables, spirulina, chlorella, wheat grass and barley grass.

Probably the best herbs are milk thistle and dandelion, which strengthen the liver system and cells. Both are better taken as liquid than pills.

Best of all is magnesium and magnesium-rich foods should be eaten in plenty, remembering that alcohol and caffeine both cause the liver stress and deplete magnesium levels.

An effective, but slightly severe, gallstone remedy is included in the Appendix. This uses a mixture of Epsom Salts, olive oil and grapefruit juice to clear out the gallstones. Reports of its effectiveness abound, but it is likely to lay you low (and keep you near a toilet) for up to three days. Still, it may be the only way to break the downward spiral of fats, lactic acid and liver clogging.

Of course, the infamous coffee enema also provokes the liver to expel toxins (though not gallstones) and should be given consideration if you are serious about detoxing your liver.

CHAPTER 5
CUTTING OUT THE BAD GUYS

The formation of a cancer cell is a multi-step process and it is very unusual for all the steps (usually thought to be six) to happen simultaneously.

Some of the biggest and worst influences on our health and our risks of developing cancer lie outside of our diets, yet in our everyday lives.

Smoke, diesel fumes, toxins in toiletries, cosmetics, cleaners, x-rays, EMFs, radon, asbestos, talcum powder etc, etc. This is a big subject and beyond the scope of this diet book.

However, what is clear is that our diet is capable of creating a negative environment that weakens and leaves us more exposed to these external factors, which can literally provide the final step and 'tip us over the edge' to cancer.

Whilst *The Tree of Life* is a diet of addition, it is worth noting that some things are at least worth trying to avoid. For example:

Dairy

We have already talked about dairy. Of the many criticisms, here are just a few:

- The average dairy cow in the USA now produces 50 (yes 50) times the volume of milk than its predecessors 20 years ago. How? Through hormones, drugs, genetic changes and super feeds which are often based on animal protein even though cows are herbivores.
- Dairy contains Insulin-like Growth Factor (IGF-1) which has been conclusively shown to cause cancer cell proliferation and has been linked in various cancers (NCI). Swedish research, for example, directly linked dairy volume consumed with prostate cancer risk levels.
- Despite the fact that Mosanto and the FDA in the USA claim IGF-1 does not cross in any volume from the gut into the bloodstream, Japanese tests with mice seem to indicate otherwise.

- The milk fats are likely to bring with them, all manner of hormones (natural and injected), antibiotics, toxins, pesticides and herbicides from the fields.
- Even with organic milk products there is a problem with human digestion, and a debate about allergies and intolerances.
- The milk of cows is designed to grow a calf to full size in less than a year, and it contains the nourishment to do it. Our human 'calves' grow to full size in sixteen or so years and rely on a different balance of hormones and nourishment.
- The high levels of fat and protein in milk prevent absorption of elements like zinc, crucial to vitamin C absorption and the fight against prostate cancer. Dairy protein actually prevents the absorption of calcium, even though dairy contains large quantities, and high blood calcium levels interfere with vitamin D levels. There is increasing evidence that vitamin D can help with cases of colon and other cancers.
- Dairy consumption also depresses magnesium and potassium levels as we saw in Chapter 3.

Dairy (and its by-products and sugars, like casein and lactose) is everywhere, and hard to avoid. Patients fighting cancer do not need high levels of protein and fat in their diets as cancer cells thrive on fat and protein. You should try to cut it out. A little goat's cheese might be alright as we have been eating this for longer than cow's cheese and it is more easily digested. But do not switch your large volume of milk consumption directly for a large volume of soya. Dr Max Gerson with his organic fruit and vegetable therapy was against soya consumption for cancer patients simply because of the fat and protein content. Cut back – use moderate soya, and rice milk.

Fat

In the Western world, we have two problems with **fats and oils:** we consume too much of them, and we largely consume the wrong sort!

Firstly, fat is anyway very high in **calories**:

1 gram protein = 4 calories,
1 gram of carbohydrate = 4 calories
1 gram fat = 9 calories.

It is not just carbohydrate that gives us energy and makes demands on insulin levels. In the USA people regularly consume 50 per cent of their calories as fat, whereas in rural China this figure can be below 10 per cent. Fats and oils are basically the same thing; fat is the solid state, oil is the liquid state. Virtually all fats and oils, when ingested, drive up oestrogen levels. (Fats produce steroids, the precursors of oestrogen.) As we will see later, oestrogen 'drives' many cancers. We noted earlier that animals on restricted calorie diets lived longer. In fact, research on rats has shown that restriction in calories stops all tumour growth.

Secondly, the majority of fats we consume (and especially the ones our children consume) are bad for us:

Saturated fats and hydrogenated vegetable oils

For many people the great majority of fats and oils consumed are saturated fat. For some people, saturated fat is virtually the only fat consumed. Junk food, fast food, chicken nuggets, onion rings, bagged snacks, crisps, salted roasted peanuts, processed foods; the list is endless. Animal fat (meat, eggs, cheese, dairy) is also a large source of saturated fat. In excess, saturated fats are difficult to metabolise, they lead to narrowing of the arteries and are linked to cancer.

The end product of their digestion, just as with smoking, is free radicals. These molecules are incomplete; they have a missing piece and are quite happy to rip the replacement from any molecule they come across, making this molecule incomplete. This in turn, rips pieces off other molecules until it is the DNA or its perfect copy messages that are attacked resulting in erroneous signals being produced. And that increases your risk of cancer – enormously.

Possibly the worst offender is the modern 'vegetable oil'. Seemingly harmless in name, these oils are often well known and have been used for centuries all over the world. However, the food companies have now refined these so that they do not spoil.

By taking them to very high temperatures, the nutrition that was present in the seed or vegetable is lost. Worse, the refining process can use gasoline, ethylene, methylchloride and chlorination, taking any last goodness out and leaving chemical traces in. Finally, in many cases the cheap oils are hydrogenated; or may be pressed and reheated to make 'vegetable oil' margarines.

In the bloodstream these are nutritionally worthless and release copious toxins and free radicals. No one is safe.

Always observe two rules:

(i) Never eat fried food; especially out of home.
(ii) Only ever use pure oils (olive, walnut, sunflower) ideally where you know the source who made them.

Polyunsaturated fats

These are a little better. Many 'safer' margarines were launched on this platform. The list includes soybean, sunflower and safflower oils. But again you must be very sure they haven't been through the processing and refining drain. Polyunsaturated oils render vitamins like beta-carotene inert.

Monounsaturated fats

The 'healthiest' oils are the monounsaturated ones: olive, flaxseed, linseed and walnut oils are the most notable. Beware the claims of margarines with these oils and names; (only very rarely, if ever, do they contain 100 per cent of these oils), and look for non-hydrogenated versions.

Again ideally choose these oils from a known supplier and in an untreated state. Oils high in monounsaturates are better for cooking as they have a high oxidation threshold and they remain stable on heating – so they do not become hydrogenated or saturated easily.

You should observe some simple rules on your 'eat to beat cancer' diet.

- Ideally reduce total fat consumption to 15–25 per cent of total daily calorie intake.
- Aim to eliminate all saturated fat from your diet.
- If buying margarine, choose brands without hydrogenated fats.

- Aim to eat most of your fat from foods or unrefined, organic oils, rich in EFAs – especially omega 3.
- If buying oil, ideally choose mechanically pressed, unrefined, organic oils in glass bottles.

Refined foods, processed foods and preserved foods

Refined foods have lost almost all their nutrients and fibre. Used in processed foods, along with chemicals, sugar and salt, E numbers and other additives, the consumer is getting little other than nutritionally empty, moderately toxic calories.

Meat products do not even need labelling on their full toxic, hormonal or additive content, so the drugs and chemicals used to fatten the animal go unmentioned.

Nitrates are frequently added to brighten the meat. In fact sodium nitrite and nitrate are widely used in dried meats, bacon, pepperoni, sausages, hams and hot dogs. Children who consume more than a dozen hot dogs a month have a considerably higher (9.5 times) risk of leukaemia. Pregnant mothers eating these foods during pregnancy have a higher incidence of brain cancer in their children.

Pickling is linked to stomach and throat cancers (the Japanese eat a lot of pickled foods). Smoked meats and fish are also linked to stomach cancer.

But preservatives abound. In 1995 Americans consumed ten pounds per year of preservatives. Britain is not far behind. Many different chemicals are used as preservatives, and yet no-one knows what effect this mix has on our bodies, and many of these chemicals have the ability to stay in our tissues for long periods of time.

A French friend telling me about road accidents in France said that exhumed bodies were hardly decomposed two years after death, such was our exposure to chemical preservatives!

Sugar

Sugar abounds in our diets and is detrimental to our entire endocrine system. There is little need to ingest sugar if you can help it. The problem is sometimes people do not know it is there, or they don't realise just how much is there.

In breakfast cereals, sucrose, corn sugar and honey are still 'sugar'; in ketchup you have more sugar than is in ice cream, which anyway has a lot; fizzy soft drinks have up to 10 spoonsful per can; 'healthy' Ribena has even more, and so on.

Anything with an 'ose' (for example: fructose, sucrose) on the label is a sugar, and may be just a nutritionally deficient source of empty calories.

Sugar also significantly weakens your immune system. How and why will be covered in Part II.

Caffeine

Caffeine depletes the body of vitamins, especially B vitamins, essential for the correct division of cells. It also depletes potassium in the body. It is a poison and has a negative effect on the immune system and on magnesium levels.

Sweeteners

Saccharin was linked to ovarian cancer, but was recently cleared, while Aspartame is being studied by SDRT, the UK brain tumour charity, for possible links to child brain tumours. In the USA, the Cancer Prevention Coalition has already pronounced against Aspartame. In America child brain tumours have recently overtaken leukaemia as the most common cancer in children.

Acrylamides

Panic set in early in 2002 when a Swedish scientist looking at whether toxins might be passing from plastic packaging into foods instead discovered highly toxic acrylamides present in chips (especially overly cooked ones), crisps and potato-bagged snacks, branded breakfast cereals, biscuits, crispbreads and crackers. Seemingly any oven-baked processed foods where the temperature was taken over 120°c were liable to be contaminated.

The World Health Organisation says that the safe limit for acrylamides is zero, such is their concern. They immediately called together 26 of the world's top scientists to develop a viewpoint and some 'solutions'. Despite the severity of the findings no hard action has been taken. Indeed a recent study announced in January 2003 by Cancer Research UK attempted to say that the levels found in these foods were not found to cause 'long term' problems. Readers are nevertheless encouraged to exert caution as the findings came from a study lasting barely three months!

For those concerned about acrylamides, two eat to beat cancer tips are:

If you like to **snack**, make your own – put out a bowl of organic sunflower, pumpkin and sesame seeds, with a few chopped nuts.

If you want a good **breakfast cereal** make your own with oats (unrefined), millet, chopped nuts, dried fruits, seeds, a little soya milk, rice milk or even water.

Eating 'out of home'

This may seem an odd inclusion, but not after you have given it some thought.

Some fast food chains only fry their food; some chains only microwave all their meals. Many restaurants will keep certain meats and fish in the freezer and microwave it to defrost it and avoid wastage. Microwaved food is genetically modified food. After exciting the electrons in the food atoms using a microwave, it is virtually impossible to have all the electrons in their original orbits. Kirlian photographs show microwaved food denuded of its natural energy and William Kopp has gathered together extensive German and Russian research. This shows that microwaved food is nutritionally deficient, and the number of cancer and precancer cells circulating in the bloodstream rises after a mircowaved meal.

Far Eastern food is little better. The Chinese food in the UK is often greasy and oily with monosodium glutamate and sugar widely used. You can get 6–10 gms of salt from one meal! Much of the dish Pad Thai is carbohydrate and oil in the UK and nothing like the meal in Thailand.

Restaurants rarely use organic ingredients, and only those 'freshly' supplied by the supermarket! Refined pasta, sugar and salt and dairy-laden sauces abound. It's a minefield for someone concerned about the quality of what they put into their body.

High cholesterol

High cholesterol causes stagnation of the whole metabolic system and it specifically inhibits the ability of the liver to detoxify the blood and therefore the tissues. High cholesterol may be caused for three reasons. You eat too much of it; you form too much of it in the body from other ingredients; you fail to expel it via the liver.

Apart from reducing your cholesterol intake (eggs, butter, lobster, liver, cheese etc.), you can prevent inhibition of the detoxing system by avoiding excess oestrogen (especially HRT and the contraceptive pill – see Chapter 7).

Meanwhile certain nutritional factors can help reduce your liver cholesterol levels: magnesium, vitamins C, B-12 and B-6, plus lecithin (choline, inositol, linoleic acid).

CHAPTER 6

THE PRINCIPLES OF HEALTHY EATING AND CANCER

Before we start to develop a healthy eating plan, let us look at some other already established views on what healthy eating means in either a preventative or corrective sense. The important thing is to learn sensible values long before you might have cancer. If you have cancer, review the information in this book carefully and slowly. Psychotherapist Rollo May concluded, *"It is an old ironic habit of human beings to run faster when we have lost our way."* Before you do anything, find your way.

(a) The Macrobiotic Diet

Some argue that this established, hundred-year-old viewpoint places too much emphasis on cooked rather than raw foods. However, it is worth a brief review for the important principles behind it.

Unlike most modern-day diets, many of which give the feeling of having been created or invented often with slimming in mind, macrobiotics is best described by the phrase 'back to basics'.

The term itself comes from the Greek: *macro* meaning great or long and *biotic* meaning, concerning life. The original word was attributed to Hippocrates, the father of modern medicine. However the concept of macrobiotics is not focussed on diet *per se* but rather the ancient Chinese belief that all life, indeed the whole universe, is a balance of two opposing forces Yin and Yang.

One's environment, one's lifestyle, one's diet and one's health are all interlinked, as is one's soul, to the greater universe and the community at large. A disease in an individual is an affliction on the community, a measure of its failings, and cannot be thought of as separate or confined to the individual.

Between 1896 and 1907 a Japanese army officer who was, even then, deeply concerned at the Westernisation of the traditional Japanese diet, implored the Japanese people to re-embrace their traditional healthy values. Sagen Ishizuka went 'back to basics' and stated his fundamental belief that the food we eat not only sustains life, it makes for our basic health and happiness. He set up a clinic and started to treat hundreds of patients with the principles of Yin and Yang, and his traditional Japanese peasant diet. His fame and success brought him the title of the 'anti-doctor'!

In the 1950s George Ohsawa brought the macrobiotic principles and diet to the West. Michio Kushi consolidated this and there is a Kushi Institute in London.

The modern macrobiotic diet is not dissimilar to the diet still used by Okinawans. Surrounded by a coral sea, their diet has less carbohydrate (and therefore calories) than even the Japanese diet, and small amounts of protein from fish and vegetables. They have an extremely high organic mineral intake, the lowest cancer rates in the world bar none, and an average life expectancy of 81.2 years, the highest in the world.

Yin elements in the macrobiotic diet are regarded as cold, slow, filling and weak; Yang in contrast is quick, dry and hard. Most disease, and especially cancer, is regarded as having a Yin cause. However for any individual all aspects of their life should be assessed by Yin and Yang principles, not just their diet. Any excess thought to be causing an illness can then be corrected or counterbalanced by providing foods of the opposite force.

The five basic principles are that:

- Foods are the foundation of health and happiness.
- Sodium and potassium are opposites in food, reflecting opposing Yin and Yang forces.
- Man's staple food is grain.
- Food should be unrefined, whole and natural.
- Food should be grown locally, ripe and consumed in season.

If you meet with a consultant concerning a cancer do not be surprised if he delves into everything in your past from diet to lifestyle, from illnesses to allergies.

He is likely to recommend a core diet, although it must be noted that a fundamental tenet of macrobiotics is that every one of us is an individual and one man's grain is another man's poison.

The core diet is likely to include:

- Whole grains (e.g. millet, barley, brown rice).
- Vegetables (including pulses and some fruits).
- Seaweed and sea vegetables.
- Fermented soya products (e.g. tofu, shoyu and miso soup).
- Regular consumption of oily fish.
- Monounsaturated oils.
- Japanese low caffeine green tea.

Everything needs to be fresh, whenever possible, and freshly prepared. Freshly prepared juices may be recommended, but raw food may not at the outset, as even if vegetables are only blanched, cooked foods have more 'fire', more energy. Dairy, sugar and meat are likely no-go foods. Organic food predominates and the diet may be extended to include exercise, yoga and even a little meditation.

A change to a macrobiotic diet and lifestyle has helped many people achieve a new health, and it has helped many cancer patients. It does require effort and time, but it does not have to be forever. Some people find its corrective action may only be needed for a year or so.

(b) The Gerson Therapy

The Gerson Therapy was developed by Dr Max Gerson (1881–1959) and first used in the 1920s as a treatment for an incurable form of TB, where he achieved phenomenal results. It must be understood from the outset that the Gerson Therapy is an extreme diet therapy used primarily by people who already have a chronic illness. It is however occasionally used in a preventative context.

Let us be quite clear. For many people, and particularly those for whom orthodox medicine had failed, the Gerson Therapy has been an important part of their 'cure'. *"Suffering isn't ennobling, recovery is"* (Dr Christiaan Barnard). Many people have recovered with the Gerson Therapy.

The basic idea of the Therapy is to stimulate the body's own immune defences to do what they normally do in a healthy body, whilst readjusting the balance of the molecules and atoms within the cells, returning them to levels normally found in healthy cells.

Once both parts of this Therapy are fully established the theory is that a diseased body will simply restore itself to full health. There is no doubt that this therapy has had notable successes, especially given that patients have often tried and failed with all available orthodox treatments beforehand.

In the case of cancer, diseased cells have been known to liquefy, which in itself creates a further problem. The process of breaking down tumours can be so effective that large amounts of toxins are released by the diseased cells into the bloodstream. However, the largest detoxification organ, namely the liver, is often seriously impaired when cancer is in the body and so it needs to be simultaneously cleansed and stimulated to deal with the extreme levels of toxins produced.

One method of achieving this is to stimulate the liver with up to five coffee enemas per day for a limited period, whilst using castor oil every other day. This causes the liver to expel its waste via increased levels of bile juices into the intestine.

The Therapy is arduous. A ten-hour day spent juicing plus making and using the coffee enemas is not unusual; and a period of two years to fully cleanse the body is not uncommon. The theory is that it takes a long time for the body to go through the multi-step cancer process, and so it takes an equally long time to restore it to full healthy working order.

Patients frequently experience 'healing reactions' when large amounts of toxins are released into the blood system.

Dr Max Gerson was described by Dr Albert Schweitzer as, "*one of the most eminent geniuses in medical history*". He originally published *A Cancer Therapy: Results of Fifty Cases* over fifty years ago. His work is now driven by his 80 year old daughter Charlotte, who stresses that it is applicable to a host of diseases, not merely cancer, and that even healthy people should consider a period on the Therapy from time to time merely as a precautionary detox.

The Therapy aims to provide optimum nutrition consisting of

a deliberate over abundance of minerals, enzymes and vitamins, whilst avoiding the toxic pesticides and herbicides of normal food by using only organic versions.

The basic principles of the Therapy are:

- The use of only organic food to avoid pesticide and herbicide toxins.
- No animal fat or protein in the first eight weeks. Both milk and soya are banned to avoid the body receiving fats and protein, both of which have been found to 'feed' cancer cells.
- No pulses (lentils, beans and, again, soya) to be consumed as they can prevent mineral uptake because of their phytic acid content.
- All water used for cooking or rinsing must be provided from distilled or reverse osmosis sources.
- Water must not be drunk as it dilutes the power of the juices. A little peppermint tea is allowed.
- Neither plastic nor tin foil may be used as it may contaminate food.
- The diet is limited to freshly made juices of vegetables, fruits and leaves, consumed within 20 minutes of preparation to avoid losses in enzyme effectiveness. Large quantities of raw fruit and vegetables are also consumed, along with some lightly steamed vegetables, stewed fruit, potatoes and oatmeal.
- The aim is to exclude sodium, whilst developing potassium intake. Fresh juices provide more easily absorbed and digested nutrients, whilst not taxing the bodily systems. The use of hourly juices over the length of the day also avoids calorie and, thus, insulin surges and actually limits the total number of calories consumed per day.
- Organic, in season, fresh vegetables and fruit are the ideal.

Absolutely **essential** to the diet therapy are:

Apples – raw.
Carrots – raw and lightly cooked.
Potatoes – baked, mashed or in potato salad.

Sweet potatoes – but only once per week.
Fresh fruit – grapes, cherries, mangoes, peaches, oranges, apricots, grapefruit, banana, tangerines, pears, plums, melons, papayas (pears and plums may be stewed).
Dried fruit – apricots, dates, figs, peaches, raisins, prunes.

Absolutely **forbidden** are:

All things bottled, canned, frozen, preserved, refined, salted, smoked and sulphured.
Bicarbonate of soda in food, toothpaste and mouthwashes.
Alcohol.
Salts.
Avocado – too much fatty acid.
Basil, oregano (aromatic oils can cause difficult reactions).
Berries (except red, black and whole currants).
Biscuits, cake, chocolate, cocoa.
Coffee (any sort), tea.
Cucumbers.
Fats and oils (except flaxseed).
Mushrooms.
Nuts (too much fatty acids/fats).
Peas (sulphured), lentils, beans, seeds (phytic acid/enzyme inhibitors).
Pickles.
Pineapples.
Refined flour.
Soft drinks, fizzy and fruit juices (preserved).
Soya (fat content and phytic acid).
Spices.
Sugar (including sweets).
Tap water.

Forbidden for first eight weeks: all dairy, eggs, meat and fish.

The type of juicer is also crucial. Centrifugal juicers simply do not get the full volumes of minerals, vitamins and enzymes out. Gerson recommended a heavy press juicer that involves two stages and a double press.

Of course, the Therapy is hard work. You need time to prepare the fresh juices, as they have to be drunk at their prime. Then there is the preparation and use of the coffee enemas. But as Goethe said, *"The day is of infinite length for him who knows how to appreciate and use it."*

(c) The Plaskett Therapy

Dr Lawrence Plaskett is vice chair of the UK Nutritional Cancer Therapy Trust. After a degree in biochemistry at Cambridge, a doctorate at London University and a number of years in food companies and government agencies, Dr Plaskett turned his extensive knowledge to updating the Gerson Therapy. His argument is simple: Dr Gerson was brilliant but since his death over 50 years ago much more has been learned about nutrition and biochemistry.

It is Plaskett's firmly held view that a nutritional approach to cancer should be nationally available. More fundamentally he argues that orthodox authorities are already in full acceptance that nutrients can protect against the inception of cancer[1]. And that various sources (one being the World Health Organisation) indicate that up to 60 per cent of cancers appear to have nutritional cause.

This may or may not be the case. Indeed, cancer development is a multi-step process and nutrition, or rather poor nutrition, may be a factor in virtually all cancers, even if other factors are more damaging or finally tip you over the edge.

As a biochemist he cites a multitude of research showing, for example:

- Flavenoids such as quercetin (apples and onions) stop the proliferation of cancer cells in vitro, especially if vitamin C is present (Kandaswami).
- Quercetin and genistein (a soya isoflavone) are the most potent anti-proliferating flavenoids in colon cancer (Kuo).
- Quercetin has potential in the treatment of leukaemia (Teofil).
- Catechins in green tea reduce size of human prostate and mammary tumours (Liao).

- Beta-carotene and vitamin C influence the survival of women with breast cancer (Ingram BJC 1994).
- Lycopene (tomatoes) inhibits prostate cell growth, as do beta-carotene, canthavanthin and retinoic acid. Coenzyme Q10 produces good results with breast cancers (Lockwood 1994).

Plaskett argues that many recent scientific discoveries have proven that Gerson was totally right and considerably 'ahead of his time'. His research into the latest scientific studies has supported, for example, the importance of omega 3 (from fish oils and linseed oil) as an essential element in the good health of cells; the use of coffee enemas to induce raised levels of glutathione S-transferases, the enzymes of liver detoxification; the use of high potassium in the diet and digestive enzymes to help increase absorption.

Where he feels recent studies have added to Gerson is that there is no need for castor oil, iodine and iodide, dried thyroid, liver juices and liver injections. Instead he recommends a very detailed and precise list of supplements, some of which vary according to the cancer.

Plaskett is very open and honest about what is still unknown about the particular ingredients of plants, vegetables and fruits that might be protective probably because he is such a precise man.

He cites carotenoids, flavenoids, indoles, thiocyanates, ellagic acid, curcumins and limonaids as protective but, given that there are 4000 flavenoids known to science for starters, he is honest enough to conclude that exactly which ones are the best, and how much should be taken of each is imprecise. With quercetin he adds that large quantities of onions might not be too good for the digestion or even breath, but supplements (which are available) might lack important 'assisting' micronutrients.

Plaskett included in his therapy:

- Coffee enemas (but less than Gerson).
- Fruit and vegetables (but less than Gerson).
- Potassium (as Gerson). Plus magnesium in addition to ensure that the sodium pump worked effectively.

- Linseed oil (as Gerson) but with fish oil.
- Digestive enzymes (as Gerson) but supplemented by amino acids.
- Bowel flora bacteria (not used by Gerson).
- Aloe vera (not used by Gerson). It stimulates the immune system and is a glycoprotein (see later).
- High fruit and vegetables but concentrating on specific ones backed by scientific evidence.
- Adjustment of the therapy to different cancers – e.g. the use of soya for hormonal cancers.
- The use of very specific levels of certain supplements.

His scientific studies have led him to seven areas for inclusion in his therapy:

1. Antioxidants – using vitamins E, C, curcuminoids from turmeric, coenzyme Q10, and multiple carotenoids and flavenoids.
2. Anti-proliferating agents to slow down cancer proliferation e.g. flavenoids, carotenoids, vitamin A, curcuminoids.
3. Detoxifying agents – e.g. organic sulphides from garlic, thiocyanates from brassicas and magnesium to increase glutathione levels.
4. Differentiators – to induce cancer cells to become more 'normal' e.g. bromelain (from pineapple), zinc, s-allyl cysteine (from garlic).
5. Inhibitors of metastasis – stopping cancer spreading, e.g. bromelain, soya.
6. Immune stimulation – e.g. aloe vera, bromelain, vitamins and minerals.
7. Angiogenesis inhibitors – inhibiting growth of new blood vessels needed by tumours, e.g. soya bean genistein, garlic.

The therapy is vigorously vegan. Dairy products, eggs, fish and meat are excluded. (A low protein diet has been shown to be effective against cancer (Tannenbaum).) All fried foods are avoided, as are processed foods.

Fresh vegetable intake is high, but uses only those with phytonutrients with proven anti-cancer properties e.g. garlic, cabbage, red-leaved lettuce, carrots, celery, parsnips, parsley, onions (red and green), tomato, aubergine, broccoli, cucumber, kale, cauliflower, sweet potatoes, radishes, brusselsprouts, endive, watercress, capsicum peppers.

Herbs and spices are used: liquorice, ginger, turmeric, mint, horseradish, oregano, rosemary, sage, thyme, chives, basil, mustard and tarragon (all organic); and Plaskett even provides a list of daily requirements:

Garlic	10 gms
Fresh onion	100–150 gms
Fresh tomato	200 gms
Turmeric powder	5 gms
Pulses, fresh and dried peas, lentils, chickpeas and beans	40 gms
Oats	50 gms
Brown rice	125 gms
Buckwheat, barley, fresh sweetcorn	occasionally
Potatoes, baked and boiled	freely used

No tea or coffee – but dandelion, organic Japanese green tea, rooibosch teas are allowed.
Soya is only included if the cancer is hormonal.
Nuts and seeds are avoided to minimise fat and protein intake.

Forbidden foods include:

Sugar of all kinds (including honey, syrup, jams)
Textured soya
Confectionery, chocolate
Ice cream
Fizzy soft drinks, squashes
Alcohol
Yeasts
Oxo, Marmite, Bovril

Modified foods
No fats (because they activate carcinogens) other than a limited amount of linseed oil and fish oil (both for omega 3)
Dried fruit (it contains sulphite).

Juices consist of six per day (all freshly squeezed):

1 glass of orange juice
2 glasses of leaf juice (endive, watercress, lettuce, green peppers, red cabbage)
3 glasses of apple and carrot (1:1)
Some beetroot juice is also used.

Of interest may be the future nutritional developments in hand for the Plaskett Therapy. For example:

- Brassica vegetables possess a number of anti-cancer agents. Even higher levels of some of these are found in germinating broccoli seeds.
- Some cultivations of garlic produce higher selenium levels and these bulbs have been linked with, for example, effective prevention of mammary tumours (Ip and Lisk). Garlic normally contains sulphide rather than selenium.
- Saffron has anti-cancer components crocin, picrocin and saframal.
- Shiitake mushrooms have 1:3 beta-glucan polysaccharide which has shown strong anti-cancer properties, (as do cordyceps and reishi mushrooms).
- Curcuminoids seem to exhibit more anti-cancer properties, the more research is done!
- Limonene-rich orange peel oil is also strong in anti-cancer properties although the oil may produce negatives too.

Clearly, here we are looking at a very detailed, disciplined and thoroughly prepared nutritional plan. The detail of supplements down to the exact number of milligrams is possibly more exact than the thirteen juices and supplements of Gerson.

Either way both men fervently believe that poor nutrition can cause cancer; and perfect nutrition can restore health.

We would be wise to heed both men.

There is no doubt that at first the Plaskett Therapy, like the Gerson Therapy, is hard work. But I have met many people who learn to use it whilst leading full and happy lives; the boss of a large corporation, a mother of a six-year-old daughter who works part-time. If it all seems too much at the start don't despair.

"Despair is the price one pays for setting oneself an impossible aim." (Graham Greene). If you have cancer, curing yourself through a diet therapy is certainly not an impossible aim.

PART II

HORMONES – THE DIRECTORS OF HEALTH

CHAPTER 7

OESTROGEN – THE KILLER IN OUR MIDST

A large number of cancers, both male and female, are hormonally responsive and in a great many of these cases the prime culprit is oestrogen, whether the natural hormone, its synthetic copy or chemicals that 'mimic' its action. The fact is that the 'oestrogen pool' is far larger in our bodies than ever before. And it's killing us. (See also *Oestrogen: The Killer in Our Midst*.)

Oestrogen is in fact not a single 'item'. Oestrogens include, for example, oestradiol and oestrone. Oestrogen in women is normally balanced by the hormone progesterone.

Oestrogen is known to cause and spread cancers (NCI). When oestrogen is added to cancer cells *in-vitro*, they proliferate (Dr Ana Soto, Tufts Cancer Center). Indeed Dr Soto also showed that there are a large number of chemicals widely used in toiletries, cosmetics, perfumes and household cleaners and disinfectants, that produce the same action as oestrogen with test cells. These are often termed oestrogen mimics or xeno-oestrogens. She has proven their effects are cumulative.

Oestrogen acts in a number of ways that can propagate human cancers. For example, oestrogen is known to help cancer messages bind to a receptor site on cells, thus spreading the cancer. Excess oestrogen reduces zinc levels in the body (the prostate, for example, is a store of zinc and low zinc levels are associated with increased risk of cancer); it increases cellular sodium levels creating a sodium/potassium imbalance; and it decreases cellular levels of oxygen for cancer cell formation.

Excess oestrogen is linked to cancers in both males and females from melanomas to ovarian, from prostate to colon, and even to diseases like Alzheimer's.

Oestrogen excess cause other severe negatives in the body and other diseases, for example, water retention, osteoporosis, fatigue, a weakening of the insulin control of blood sugar, memory loss, increases blood clotting and histamine levels, along with allergies, depression and dry skin! It destroys folate and biotin, both essential in DNA replication and the immune system.

Each week people ring our magazine **icon** (*Integrated Cancer and Oncology News*) to ask about breast cancers, prostate cancers, colon cancers, melanoma and even rare cancers like Hurtle's cells, all of which have been linked with high oestrogen levels. Many more cancers are linked to this same hormone.

The 'oestrogen pool' levels are increasing in our bodies for three primary reasons:

- We are making more of it ourselves – as we will see, our diets, the way we eat, being overweight and our lifestyles cause a greater production.
- We are ingesting more of it – women who take the pill or HRT; all of us who drink recycled city water, or eat animal fats.
- We are absorbing more chemicals and toxins that have a chemical composition similar to oestrogen once in the bloodstream (oestrogen mimics).

Although it is relatively easy for a woman to understand that oestrogen might be involved in her cancer, men find it hard to believe that this 'female' hormone could have anything to do with theirs. However it is clearly implicated in, for example, prostate and testicular cancers.

Let us start with the most obvious link:

Oestrogen and breast cancers

As we have said, the Bush people of the Kalahari Desert in Africa have a diet largely from vegetable sources with the odd, lean and usually small animal as a treat. Of course, they also have no stress, pollution and electro-magnetic radiation to worry about. Seven per cent of their population are over 65 years of age. They have worn but not bad teeth, whilst in some parts of Europe a third of the population has no teeth at all. They eat little or no animal fat and never dairy from cows.

And they have no breast cancer.

Breastfeeding is the norm and continues until the child is four to five years old. In the West some mothers do not breastfeed their children at all, whilst many rarely exceed six months.

In August 2002 Cancer Research UK published the definitive study on breastfeeding and breast cancer.

It concluded that **the more time a women spends breastfeeding in her life, the less her own risk of breast cancer.**

Scientists have also shown that **the fewer menstrual cycles a woman goes through in her life, the lower her chance of breast cancer.**

Scientists have long been concerned in the West about the lengthening years of fertility in women, a fact that has its roots in our diets. One hundred and fifty or more years ago a woman was likely to have been fertile from the age of 16 to her late thirties. Without contraception she may have had four children, and these she would have breastfed for nine months or more. The current New York female may have menstrual cycles lasting from her twelfth to her fiftieth birthday, and have two or less children en route. This increases her total number of periods from around 200 to as many as 440. And that's a lot more monthly oestrogen surges and resultant hormone fluctuation. Scientists believe this is also reflected in, for example, increasing incidence of endometriosis and polycystic ovary syndrome.

The Collaborative Group on Hormonal Factors in Breast Cancer, supported by Cancer Research UK, published findings in the *Lancet* in late July 2002 on 'Breast Cancer and Breastfeeding'.

Having reviewed over 50,000 women with breast cancer and 97,000 without, in 47 studies across 30 countries they concluded that the relative risk of breast cancer decreased by 7 per cent for each birth, plus 4.3 per cent for every 12 months of breastfeeding.

These figures seem to apply whether one is studying a developed, or a developing country.

In the report the main reason given for these findings confirmed that, 'the more periods a woman has, the greater her overall oestrogen production during her lifetime. Oestrogen is known to have a negative effect on the breast tissue causing it to become dense. And dense breast tissue is risky breast tissue.'

The report finished by stating that there were about 470,000 women in developed countries with breast cancer, and if women had 2.5 children on average and breastfed each for 12 months longer than they currently do, about 11 per cent (50,000) breast cancers would be prevented annually (Valerie Beal, Cancer Research UK, Epidemiology Unit).

Worse, **modern women add to their levels of oestrogen by taking the pill or HRT**. Again Cancer Research UK published data that showed women who take the pill increase their chances of breast cancer by 26 per cent. If they take it into their thirties this extra risk rises to 58 per cent. For the 10 per cent of women who take it into their 40s, the figure increases to 144 per cent.

It is worth noting that the original FDA approval for the pill was granted following a single trial on 132 Puerto Rican women, despite five of them dying during the trial (*Science* 259, 1993 Marshall). This resulted in a newer, safer pill in the 70s with a lower dose of oestrogen. However, to this day, there is no single long-term trial showing the pill to be safe.

HRT is a similar though weaker oestrogen-based pill. The late Doctor John Lee, who spent more than twenty years looking into oestrogen and its effects on the body, was clear that too much oestrogen is the essence of the problems facing women at menopause. Yet HRT, and thus more oestrogen, is prescribed to 'alleviate symptoms'!

In 2002, a seven-year HRT trial, part of the Women's Health Initiative study, was stopped in the USA, when the dangers started to emerge. The part of the 16,000 women trial involving a mixed synthetic oestrogen and progestin pill had resulted in a doubling of breast cancer risk. The part of the trial using an oestrogen-only pill was allowed to continue but 2.2 million women in the UK heard that their risk of just breast cancer rises by at least 27 per cent solely by taking oestrogen-based HRT. (The Boston Nurses Study report in 1995 contained the same 27 per cent figure for breast cancer, but went on to conclude that there was significant risk of other cancers like ovarian too.) If HRT were a herbal supplement, it would have been banned within a week. Interestingly, even the pharmaceutical companies list over 100 potential problems associated with HRT. The one thing they don't tell you is that oestrogen supplementation can be addictive. The *British Medical Bulletin* (1992: 48) states a concern for women wishing to stop HRT after long-term treatment!

Oestrogen and prostate cancer

The male hormone is testosterone and again there are several types. A precursor is progesterone. Men also make the oestrogen, oestradiol but in much, much smaller quantities. However, as we shall see it is almost impossible for men to escape the ingestion of large quantities of oestrogen and oestrogen mimics.

Testosterone and oestradiol influence each other. Oestradiol stimulates the growth of the prostate gland, but as men age their progesterone levels decline and with them their testosterone levels, leaving the oestradiol aided and abetted by all the oestrogen mimics, to cause problems. With declining progesterone a type of testosterone (DHT) is produced which actually sets off the cancer chain reaction. Oestrogen stimulates the production of DHT from testosterone (Thompson, Texas), and anti-oestrogens (for example, Finistride and ICI) can stop this (Singapore National Cancer Centre). Monash Cancer Centre in Australia has concluded that localised oestrogen is the driving force in prostate cancer, and this has been confirmed in the Concord Cancer Institute, Sydney. Men should be quite clear. Testosterone declines as you age, and it does not cause prostate cancer. Oestrogen, and particularly oestrogen mimics, turn 'safe' testosterone into very 'unsafe' DHT.

Natural progesterone

Natural progesterone in the body balances the hormone oestrogen. Whilst oestrogen declines in women at menopause to about 60 per cent of original levels, just enough to stop ovulation, progesterone falls to almost zero, a little being made by the adrenals.

In prostate cancer synthetic progestin is used to balance and neutralise the testosterone, but in reality its actual action is to balance and neutralise the oestrogen effect! Some people have suggested this is a case of "right drug, wrong reason"!

So the progestin, like the oestrogen inhibitors ICI and Finisteride, acts against the oestrogen.

Anastrozole is the new 'wonder drug' for post-menopausal women at risk from breast cancer. Its effect? To limit oestrogen production in their bodies.

But why not use something natural (and cheap) without side effects to do this job. Natural progesterone can be prescribed by certain 'integrated doctors' and is worth looking into.

Some people believe Wild Yam supplements and creams can help. Wild Yam will stimulate the adrenals and can provide the precursor raw materials to progesterone but also other hormones like oestrogen and testosterone. It is nowhere near as focussed though as taking natural progesterone.

The diet factor

Our diets and the way we eat also cause surges of oestrogen. For example:

High carbohydrate, high oestrogen

A high carbohydrate diet provides high calories, and often the calories most usually come from refined foods like white rice, bread and pasta, or from sugary drinks, like fruit juices and fizzy soft drinks, or from chocolate bars and snack products. These release their energy stores quickly, forcing insulin to be produced rapidly to prevent excess sugar in the blood reaching the brain.

Furthermore, nowadays, we tend to eat less meals but bigger ones, with high starch and high fat content both of which pile on the calories. High calorie meals cause high insulin levels. Insulin surges completely throw out the balance between all the hormones in the body and one in particular also surges – oestrogen. A 5 to 10 per cent reduction in daily calorie intake reduces oestrogen levels by 20 per cent.

Phytoestrogens and oestrogen limitation

Worse, the types of foods we eat do not help. The vegetables and pulses we ate in abundance two hundred years ago produced large amounts of phytoestrogens in our bodies. These substances, although weaker than human oestrogen, competed with it and helped control its levels. For example, in women with high ginestein levels (a phytoestrogen), menstrual cycles are elongated, more regular and reduced in number. Soya is nowadays perhaps one of the most recognised contributors of phytoestrogens but many Western vegetables and pulses used to provide them daily in our diets. Women in the Far East have blood ginestein levels up to one thousand times those of New York women. But we could have these protective levels too; there is no need to switch to soya, just remember the foods that have protected us in the UK for centuries: pulses, broad beans, lentils, peas, chickpeas, plus green vegetables, carrots, red peppers, broccoli, cabbage and herbs all increase your phytoestrogens and protective carotenoids.

In hormonally driven cancers that spread, the cancer cell messages lock onto receptor sites on cells. Oestrogen helps that process, but phytoestrogens which have a slightly different biochemical formula to human oestrogen block these adjacent receptor sites preventing any cancer spread. Professor Trevor Powles, former head of the breast cancer unit at the Royal Marsden Hospital calls them anti-oestrogens and is quite clear on their benefits. At the Royal Marsden they are researching the benefits of red clover with cancer patients. Red clover, the herb of Hippocrates, gives even better levels of certain phytoestrogens and Professor Powles is confident that they will find a level of usage that is successful with cancers.

In July 2002, Cancer Research UK published research findings on the clear benefits of soya. A study involving two new pieces of research between Cancer Research UK, The National University of Singapore and the US National Cancer Institute found that a diet rich in soya products could affect the make up of breast tissue, potentially reducing breast cancer.

Women in the Far East who consume the most soya are 60 per cent less likely to have dense breast tissue. And as we said, dense tissue is clearly associated with an increased risk of breast cancer. The study's co-author, Dr Stephen Duffy of Cancer Research UK's Mathematics, Statistics and Epidemiology Department in London says: "*There has always been a question mark over a connection between soya and breast cancer. Some studies have suggested a link but others haven't. This research shows for the first time how the amount of soya a woman eats may have an effect on breast tissue and in turn may potentially reduce her risk of breast cancer.*"

In Asian women, menopausal symptoms are almost unheard of, and they have half the levels of oestradiol and oestrone circulating in their bodies. Phytoestrogens in soya have been closely linked to lowering circulating oestradiol levels (Lee-Jane Lu).

As a result men get less prostate and women less breast and endometrial cancers. Phytoestrogens from soya and other vegetables have been shown to be especially protective in prostate cancer (*Lancet* 1993: 342).

Pesticides and oestrogens

Many pesticides and herbicides act as oestrogen mimics inside the body after ingestion. Whether we eat them directly due to their residue in our foods, or we eat the animals that ate them, hardly matters. DDT, DDE, dieldrin, lindane, methoxychlor, benzene hexachloride, kepone and more than fifty others are widely used in the world's food production and all have the ability to mimic oestrogen in the body.

The animal fat we eat brings with it both oestrogens from the animals themselves plus these oestrogen mimics from the toxins in the fields. Fat is a wonderful solvent and so toxic animal fat adds to our already high levels of oestrogen.

The mimics are hardly ever biodegradable and so enter the body and 'lock on' to cellular receptor sites interfering with a host of biochemical processes and making them hard to excrete. Such action has been associated with everything from brain deficiencies to reduced sperm counts, even cellular DNA interference (*Lancet* 1993) and folic acid depletion (Moscow Cancer Institute).

Our dairy and particularly milk consumption does not help us.

In Israel between 1975 and 1983, extremely high rates of breast cancer in very young women were found to be caused by oestrogen mimics, specifically from DDT and lindane, in dairy. A number of organochlorine pesticides were banned and the figures subsequently returned to 'normal' levels.

Water and oestrogen

One of the biggest sources of unwanted oestrogen for men and women is tap water in large cities where the water is recycled.

With millions of women on the pill and HRT relieving themselves into a city's water supplies and little attention paid to filtration of the hormone, recycled tap water has become more than a little risky. Links to male genital problems have been made in several scientific studies (for example, Athlone Institute, Ireland). The only solution is to use a top quality reverse osmosis water filter although some people frown on these, as they argue that the water emerges too pure!

Plastic bottled water doesn't help either. Indeed, plastic packaging on all drinks and foods may leach phthalates, which are also 'oestrogen mimics', into the food and drink in varying quantities. Dr Ana Soto once famously observed her cancer cells growing because phthalates were leaching from the plastic dishes into her cell cultures!

Oestrogen in the home

Although beyond the scope of this diet book, it is worth noting here that oestrogen mimics surround us. The average American woman has a toxin level in her bloodstream four times that of her male equivalent!

Cosmetics, from face creams to lipsticks, can all contain oestrogen mimics. Sodium lauryl sulphate in soaps, bubble bath, shampoos etc can increase the permeability of the skin by up to 40 per cent. This just allows more mimics to pass into the bloodstream. In December 2002, Swedish researchers showed that three quarters of perfumed toiletry products tested contained phthalates and in particular DEHP. Perfumes, perfumed body sprays, hairsprays and hair products were the main culprits. With pregnant women, these have been linked to reproductive health problems in male offspring, including undescended testicles, smaller organ size and even to increased levels of testicular cancer.

In a German study, endometriosis was linked to chemicals called PCBs and cases of vaginal and cervical cancers have been linked to nonylphenols, which are oestrogen mimics often used in spermicides and contraceptive jellies.

Clearly men are not immune from this – they wash their faces with soap, use perfumed shaving foam and aftershave or perfumed sprays and deodorants everyday.

It's easy to see how we increase our 'oestrogen pool levels'. Men and women should ensure that they find a reputable provider of carcinogen-free products for their cosmetic, toiletry and bathroom needs. In our travels we have found one company that seems to do this; the only company recommended in the USA by the Cancer Prevention Coalition – Neways.

But it doesn't end there. Volatile organic carbons can be ingested, for example, by breathing the petrol fumes while filling the car; or from inks in fax machines or computer circuitry if your office is not properly ventilated. Dyes and glues have also been known as the source of these oestrogen mimics.

One of the biggest sources is cleaning products; from washing-up liquids to spray cleaners (for furniture or bathrooms), to detergents and polishes. No wonder that women who work at home have 40 per cent more toxins in their bloodstreams than their sisters who go out to work! Recent work by Soto has shown these 'mimics' to be cumulative. The only advicc is to find a supplier of toxin-free products. Again we, like CPC USA, recommend Neways.

So, as you can see there is both a direct and an indirect link between our lifestyles, our diets and our oestrogen levels – and oestrogen is implicated in many cancers and much ill health.

In summary

- Do everything you can to kick the oestrogen out of your life.
- Do not take the pill or HRT; don't drink cow's milk and avoid dairy as much as possible.
- Eat more pulses and a little soya.
- Buy a reverse osmosis filter and clean up your water.
- Use in-home cleaners, toiletries and cosmetics that come from a reputable, toxin-free supplier.
- Go organic where possible to reduce oestrogen mimics in pesticides and herbicides.
- Consult an integrated doctor about the use of natural progesterone.

For more information whether you are male or female and interested in melanoma to prostate, or colon to brain cancer, read

Oestrogen: The Killer in Our Midst. (Details can be found at the back of this book.)

CHAPTER 8

EICOSANOIDS – CONTROLLING THE WELL-BEING OF YOUR CELLS

In 2000, the Mayo Clinic published results which showed that small daily amounts of aspirin (81 mgs) and omega 3 would reduce the risk of prostate cancer by 40 per cent. This was not the first such indication. Both omega 3 and aspirin had previously been linked to reduction in colon, bowel, lung and pancreatic cancer risk. These results keep repeating themselves. For example, in February 2003 US scientists published a report in the medical journal, *Gastroenterology*, suggesting that aspirin cut risks of cancer of the gullet by 50 per cent. In April 2003 there was a US desk study confirming daily aspirin prevents breast cancer. In May 2004 Cancer Research UK were making headline news with 'an aspirin a day can slash the risk of developing breast cancer by almost a third'.

As I was writing an article on prostate cancer, I rang a UK charity for a view on the Mayo clinic's findings. The nurses on the 'helpline' had no knowledge of these findings saying that they did not like to recommend aspirin, and anyway the results were new and unconfirmed.

In 1982 John Vane won a Nobel Prize, a knighthood and a lot of money for his work on eicosanoids. He was particularly interested in one group of eicosanoids called prostaglandins, and concluded, even then, that they were reduced by the effect of aspirin. So the Mayo Clinic research is hardly 'new research'!

Many people believe hormones are made solely in the endocrine glands. In fact the largest volume of hormones produced are the eicosanoids, very short-lived hormones lasting less than a couple of seconds and produced by the nuclear envelope in every cell in your body.

There are over a hundred eicosanoids, each producing different responses; some helpful, some negative. The nuclear envelope is stimulated by external chemicals to produce any or all of these, 'good' or 'bad', thus changing the environment of the cell, and with it the risk of, for example, inflammation or cancer. Worse, some eicosanoids like prostoglandins are helpful in small quantities but in excess cause significant problems around cells and in tissues. Thus it is important to try to keep their levels of production regular. Hormones are very powerful chemicals with only very small amounts needed to bring dramatic changes.

This has huge implications for your health. For example, it has been clearly established that depression is linked with increased rates of cancer. A depressed brain sends out signals through the nervous system and the endocrine system to every cell in your body. The depression signals reach the nuclear envelope and stimulate localised negative hormones – a depressed brain makes for depressed prostate cells too!

Depression produces a lowered oxygen-carrying capacity in the blood, often up to 30 per cent. And since oxygen is the enemy of cancer, depression allows cancer to thrive.

Stress is known to work in much the same way. A stressed brain stimulates the adrenals to produce cortisol. Cortisol then stimulates an enzyme on the cell's nuclear envelope to produce negative local eicosanoids. A stressed brain makes for stressed breast cells.

Eicosanoids and diet

Whilst drugs and internal chemicals like steroids and cortisol have this negative effect on localised eicosanoid production so too do other natural bodily chemicals, the most relevant to your eating habits being **insulin.**

First let us look at how eicosanoids are made. Basically all the fats and oils you eat, whether they are animal fats, fish oils, nut oils or fast food cooking oils collect in a pool, which we will call the fatty acid pool. This pool provides the raw ingredients for the synthesis of eicosanoids 'good' or 'bad'. However, the production of bad eicosanoids requires an enzyme to cause the chemical chain reaction. This enzyme is turned on and stimulated by such chemicals as steroids, cortisol and insulin. Thus large meals, high carbohydrate meals, excess sugar or sudden bursts of sweetened soft drinks or fruit juices will all cause insulin surges which stimulate the enzyme and turn the environment of your cells negative, significantly increasing the risk of cancer and other illnesses.

Steroids, cortisol and insulin amongst other chemicals thus increase your risk of cancer. Nowhere is this more acute than in your colon where a highly toxic bile acid is stimulated by excesses of fats and alcohol – lithocholic acid is produced after a similar enzyme to the one above is stimulated.

But as various research studies have found, there are elements of your diet that can be highly protective. For example, vitamin D has been found to detoxify lithocholic acid (Howard Hayes Medical Unit, May 2002). In normal cells and in the colon example, omega 3 and aspirin will turn off this negative enzyme causing less of the negative eicosanoids to be made and allowing more of the favourable ones to be produced. Hence their role in reducing risk of cancer. Importantly both ginger and garlic also contain substances which will turn off the same enzyme and help reduce the toxins in the cellular environment. One thing is increasingly clear. Inflammation is being acknowledged more and more as a precursor to cancer and there are a number of simple ways you can protect yourself.

In summary

- The best source of omega 3 is fish oils, which provide long-chain omega 3. It would further appear that only long-chain omega 3 has this protective effect; short-chain omega 3 from seed oils like flaxseed and linseed seems inert. Flaxseed and linseed omega 3 can convert to long-chain omega 3, however it is worth noting that in the first half of the twentieth century fish oil production was regularly 75,000 tonnes per annum; now it is just 20,000. Sadly, we are consuming less fish and far less protective fish oils.
- You can take a small dose of aspirin each day (the Mayo Clinic recommended 81 mgs). Of course you don't have to take aspirin. Foods like aloe vera, contain salicylate, and almonds will have a similar but natural analgesic effect. Natural aspirin can be found as willow bark.
- So there you have the first example of how a few foods, for

example, garlic, ginger, oily fish and aloe vera can actually protect you and the localized environment to the cells in your body. From prostate cells to colon cells. Eat to beat cancer in action!

CHAPTER 9

INSULIN – THE BITTER-SWEET HORMONE

So, as we have seen, insulin can stimulate both oestrogen production and 'bad' eicosanoid production – and both of these increase the risk of cancer.

Diabetes

By far the biggest issue with insulin is that of diabetes. An understanding of diabetes and factors that cause high insulin production is necessary to help plan a healthy diet.

The source of insulin is the pancreas, an organ also suspected by many to play a huge role in the control of both stem cells and cancer cells.

When your mother's egg and father's sperm fuse, the resultant cell multiplies extremely rapidly. Around day 56 these first cells, or stem cells, differentiate into eye, ear and toe cells. And these cells divide at a more normal rate. The organ that causes this switch from stem cells to differentiated cells is the pancreas. Cancer cells resemble stem cells. They too are undifferentiated, and they too multiply rapidly.

The pancreas makes two hormones: **insulin**, which takes sugar out of the bloodstream and stores it in the liver, muscles or fat cells when blood sugar levels are too high, and **glucagon**, which responds to low blood sugar levels by causing stored glucose to be released.

There are two basic types of diabetes. Type 1, which can be hereditary but can also occur after viral infection. Type 1 diabetes sees permanent damage to the insulin producing cells in the pancreas. Artificial insulin must be given to sufferers or they will go into a sugar-induced coma.

Type 2, or late onset diabetes, seems to be brought on exclusively by our modern diet typically when people are in their fifties. Indeed it is not so 'late onset' these days with more and more adolescents and children succumbing to it.

Mississippi is the worst region in the USA for late onset diabetes.

In 2002 the rate had increased to 8 per cent of adults. The health authorities blamed the high level of fried food in the diet.

However the figures for diabetes are expected to double by 2010 (*British Journal of Community Nursing* 2002: 7). Whilst in 1982 about 4 per cent of children (under 12s) in the USA had diabetes, by 1994 the figure had risen to 16 per cent!

Even in the UK the growth rate of diabetes in under-fives is currently running at 11 per cent per annum (*BMJ* 1997: 315).

Late onset diabetes has been simplistically linked to calorie intake, but is increasingly thought to be caused by a complex mixture of a number of factors like high carbohydrate/sugar intake, being overweight, high intake of hydrogenated fats (also called trans fatty acids) and even milk consumption as we shall see.

The causes of diabetes – a modern diet

A French scientist, Dr Michel Montignac, developed a theory about the disease in the eighties which, although largely ignored at the time, is now being given credence.

Back in the seventies, scientists thought that all overweight people suffered from overproduction of insulin when ingesting carbohydrates, resulting in a storing of the sugars, as fat. Montignac felt it was not obesity that was causing the diabetes but simply an overworked, exhausted pancreas.

By 1997 the Harvard School of Public Health had researched 65,000 women and concluded that the ones who developed diabetes most commonly ate a low fibre diet, which was also high in refined/empty sugars. (*JAMA* 1997: 277). A second study of 40,000 men supported this (*Diabetes Care* 1997: 20).

These findings caused a switch from the theory that a sedentary lifestyle, obesity and stress were causing the problems, pointing the finger of blame firmly at the intake of nutritionally ‘empty’ sugars and carbohydrate, i.e. a modern Western diet.

When the Harvard study also found that hydrogenated vegetable oils could bring on diabetes (*American Journal of Clinical Nutrition* 2001: 273) researchers started to understand why the disease was booming in the young. Hydrogenated vegetable oils are commonly in fast foods and processed foods.

Another surprising contributor was then found to be cow’s milk, which anyway contains insulin-like stimulators (IGF1) as we saw in Chapter 7. Finnish research (Diabetes 2000:49) concluded that children had a five-fold increase in diabetes if fed cow's milk during infancy. Mothers, your babies need to eat to beat cancer too: breast is best!

Other factors linked to diabetes have been vaccines, beta-blockers and antidepressants like Prozac. Interestingly the *Journal of Cardiovascular Risk* carried an article at the start of 2003 linking red wine consumption with protection against diabetes. I'll drink to that!

The ingestion of refined carbohydrates and sugars

Insulin is produced in response to increases in blood sugar levels to protect our brains from damage by excess blood sugar. Any sugars entering the bloodstream are invariably taken straight to the heart and brain. Sugar has been 'refined' for over two hundred years in an attempt to prevent it decomposing. It is now 96 per cent sucrose and can create a drug-like dependency in the body. Withdrawal symptoms are common in people who cut sugar from their diets. It also depletes the body of calcium. Corn syrup has similar problems and it depletes the body of B vitamins.

Our damaging eating habits are worsening. Just look at our diets. Carbohydrate-rich, processed breakfast cereals, processed fruit juice (which is little more than sugared water anyway!), sugar in tea or coffee, waffles, hash browns and fried, calorie-heavy ham and eggs – and that's just the average American breakfast available at drive-ins for less than $7. No wonder obesity is running at 26 per cent. Sixty per cent of 16-year-old boys in the USA are overweight or obese. It's getting worse and the figures show that the UK is not far behind with adult obesity at 21 per cent.

Snack food is sugar and hydrogenated oil rich. Consider empty calorie soft drinks, where a fizzy soft drink may contain ten spoonsful of sugar; or chocolate, buns, cakes, pasta, ready meals, breakfast cereal, cheesecake and biscuits. Then you have an endless list of high street fast food outlets from burger to pizza 'restaurants'.

The average individual will consume over 170 lbs of sugar per year (Beasley, *The Betrayal of Health)*. Processed and preserved foods are the main culprits as the sugar is hidden.

Ladies who lunch may have a penchant for a slimming pasta and a glass of Chardonnay. Whole grains for thousand of years provided fibre, protein, amino acids and essential B vitamins. No longer are whole grains ever on the menu. Refined pasta is no longer a living food. It has lost 80 per cent of its vitamins, 90 per cent of its minerals and almost 100 per cent of its fibre. Oh, and by the way ladies, its calorie levels have increased by about 10 per cent per gram. Nutritionally empty and higher calories, how healthy is that?

Natural fibre seems to have been forgotten in all this. Instead we take supplements or harsh, enriched bran additives. Natural cellular membrane fibre slows down the rate of release of sugar from inside the cells. Adding bran fibre to the diet cannot achieve this. Furthermore, many natural fibres, apart from aiding our excretion processes and bowel movements, can even bind to and neutralise fats in the bloodstream. This defence mechanism has been lost with refining.

Big meals, insulin rushes

It is not just the types of food that we eat that cause surges; it is the way we eat.

Skipping breakfast has become the norm for many people, leaving the 'need' for a large lunch and a big evening meal.

But fat is also calorie rich, and these high fat, high carbohydrate, highly refined large meals just flood the system with sugar, causing great stress on the pancreas.

Glycaemic index

The refining process for grains, rice, processed meals and oils has a lot to answer for. Montignac went on to develop a diet or slimming plan. His basic recommendation was, "eat as much as you like but always foods with a **low glycaemic index** (GI)."

Sugar or glucose is the benchmark with a GI of 100. Refined foods which lack fibre, and over cooked foods, where the fibre (or cellulose walls of vegetables) has broken down, have GIs approaching 100 meaning a sudden rush of sugar into the bloodstream and an overworked pancreas. Foods like jasmine rice (109) or rice cakes (82) are typical of this.

It is also why raw fruit and vegetables are so beneficial, as their intact fibre aids a slower and controlled sugar release process.

All foods can be assigned a GI but this only measures their

'quality' in terms of sugar release. It needs to be coupled with their 'quantity'. Thus glycaemic load (which is what really troubles the pancreas) is the multiple of the two.

Thus spaghetti (150 gms) when cooked has 48 gms of carbohydrate and a GI of 44. Hence the glycaemic load is 44 x 48 ÷ 100 = 21. So, when looking at the figures below, think also of the amounts you will consume.

Meats and fish have GIs of zero. Fresh, raw vegetables are usually 10 or below unless root crops. Fruits and nuts are usually in the 10–30 spread. Green vegetables around 15, pulses around 30. Cooking takes carrots from 20 to 40.

GI foods – some examples:

Food	GI
Apple, raw	38
Apple juice	40
Apricots, raw	57
Apricots, dried	30
Banana, raw	52
Barley, boiled	25
Basmati white rice	58
Broad beans	79
Buckwheat, boiled	54
Bulgar, boiled	48
Carrots, boiled	41
Chickpeas, boiled	28
Cereals, unrefined	40
Cereals, refined	75
Coco Pops	70
Croissant	67
Fish fingers	38
Gluten-free muesli	39
Ice cream	65
Kidney beans	52
Kiwi fruit, raw	58
Lentils, boiled	30
Lychees, canned	79
Milk, fresh	31
Millet, boiled	71
Muesli bar	61
Mung beans	39
Noodles, fresh	40
Oats	49
Orange	42
Orange juice	53
Parsnips	97
Peach, fresh	42
Peach, canned	58
Pear	38
Pecans, raw	10
Oat porridge, whole	55
Potato crisps	54
Raisins	64
Rice noodles	40
Ryvita	69
Soya milk	36
Soya beans	14
Strawberries	40
Sweetcorn	46
Sweet potato	44
Wholemeal bread	71
Yam	37
Yoghurt, low fat	38

It is interesting to note that the Bush people of the Kalahari and of Australia have their staple diet carbohydrates (e.g. Aboriginals use flour from the wattle seed) with GIs of only 10. Whole grains in our diet are beneficial and protective. The second you refine them, the benefits disappear and they have a negative effect.

Low GI foods:

- Lead to lower insulin levels and rejuvenate a stressed pancreas,
- Help lower blood fats and cholesterol,
- Reduce risk of diabetes and heart disease,
- Reduce risk of cancer and improve overall health.

In summary

- We need to refocus our diets.
- We must eat less calories than we think we need. We must eat more but smaller meals, for example, six per day.
- We must eat whole grain, unrefined products, pulses and nuts with a low glycaemic index to avoid the insulin rush. And eat more fresh and raw vegetables and fruit where the sugar is slowly released as the fibre breaks down.
- We must avoid all unnecessary and nutritionally empty, low fibre sugar; in fizzy drinks, beers, puddings, snacks and hidden in ready-meals and processed foods.
- If your insulin does go out of control, you are on your way to diabetes or cancer, or both. Beware.

If you want to eat to beat cancer follow these simple suggestions:

- Make your own breakfast muesli with whole grain, dried fruits, nuts and seeds. Make your own fresh fruit juices or better still eat a plate of whole fruit and let the fibre take care of you. Get your day off to a healthy start.
- Eat smaller meals, more frequently. Graze, don't pig.
- Learn to control your own insulin, by learning to cut out sugars and empty calories, whilst vowing never to have a meal without natural fibre or whole grains on your plate or in your bowl. If a carbohydrate is refined, don't eat it.
- A three- to five-day raw vegetable and fruit diet (or similar juices) may well help to rejuvenate your pancreas.

CHAPTER 10

HELPING THE BODY'S HELPERS!

Hormones that might help

Three hormones have been especially indicated in cancer prevention activities: melatonin, human growth hormone and DHEA.

All three peak in production terms in our bodies around the age of sixteen. They then fall away to almost zero in our fifties. Albert Einstein was being philosophical when he opinioned *"The tragedy of life is what dies inside a man when he lives."* But he could have been talking about these three essential hormones.

Melatonin stimulates the thymus gland to produce cells which seek and destroy rogue cells. It is also a know antioxidant and free radical neutraliser, and has been shown to depress oestrogen levels. Women whose sleep patterns are disrupted (for example, night shift workers) have lowered melatonin levels and an increased rate of breast cancers.

The amino acid tryptophan is the precursor of serotonin, which in turn is the precursor of melatonin. Tryptophan is an essential amino acid (i.e. you have to eat it – you cannot make it). To eat to beat cancer find it in all protein-rich foods. Best sources for you would be lean turkey, fish, bananas, dried dates and peanuts.

Tryptophan works best if ingested about two hours before going to sleep. It will have a 'relaxing' effect. Tryptophan can be used by the brain along with magnesium, vitamin B6 and niacin to produce serotonin. About one and a half hours after you fall asleep, melatonin kicks in to promote a deeper sleep. If tryptophan is taken as a supplement, a balanced B complex pill should be taken as well.

You can take a melatonin supplement. They are easily obtained in the USA, but in the UK are only available on prescription. Levels of 3–6 mgs are usually taken but levels of 10 mgs and above have been known to cause hallucinations.

Human growth hormone (Hgh) is also produced about ninety minutes after falling asleep, and its production also peaks at puberty, to decline to almost zero in the fifties. Hgh can be stimulated by resistance training at almost any age when the muscles are overworked and 'tear' slightly.

Hgh helps mobilise and burn fats and stimulates the conversion of protein into lean muscle. Most importantly it also stimulates the production of the seek-and-destroy immune cells.

Even after fifty years of age, diet can restimulate Hgh production. The amino acids argenine, tyrosine and ornithine will stimulate its production, but in fact there is a whole set of amino acids and vitamins and minerals required for best results (argenine, tyrosine, ornithine, tryptophan and glycine work synergistically with vitamins like the B vitamins, vitamin C and minerals zinc, calcium, magnesium and potassium).

Argenine in found in nuts, brown rice, oatmeal, raisins, seeds, meats and wholemeal bread. It is interchangeable in the body with ornithine. Argenine production (from the pituitary) ceases in adults around the age of thirty. Trauma will also stop its production.

It is interesting to note that calorie restriction limits insulin production and also stimulates Hgh production, having the double benefit of controlling negative hormones whilst aiding the levels of this significant cancer fighter.

DHEA (dehydroepiandrosterone) is a natural hormone produced by the adrenal glands. Again its production declines with age. It is protective against free radicals and some people use DHEA supplements although results are very mixed and some cancer risks have been noted. It seems to be weakened by oestrogen and stimulated by progesterone. Wild yam acts as a precursor and natural stimulator of DHEA (as for progesterone), and has also been shown to be an excellent booster of the immune system.

SECTION B

THE TREE OF LIFE

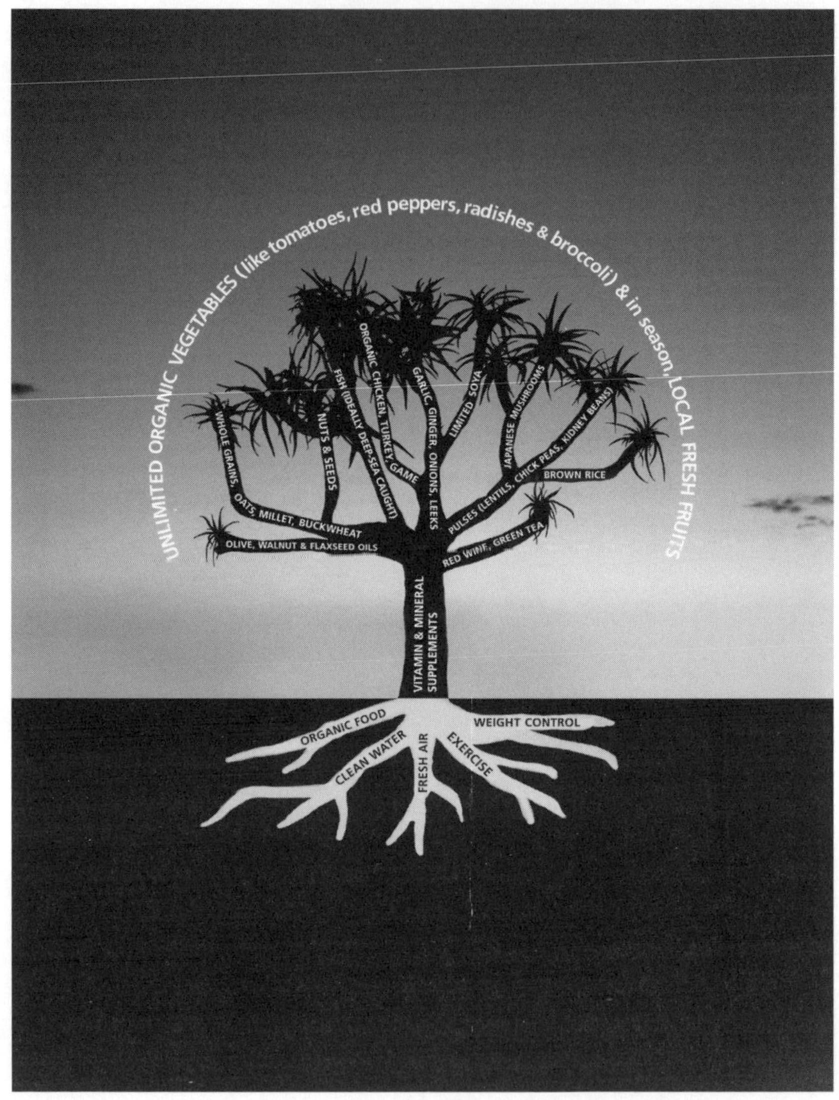
UNLIMITED ORGANIC VEGETABLES (like tomatoes, red peppers, radishes & broccoli) & in season, LOCAL FRESH FRUITS
WHOLE GRAINS, OATS, MILLET, BUCKWHEAT
OLIVE, WALNUT & FLAXSEED OILS
NUTS & SEEDS
FISH (IDEALLY DEEP-SEA CAUGHT)
ORGANIC CHICKEN, TURKEY, GAME
GARLIC, GINGER, ONIONS, LEEKS
LIMITED SOYA
JAPANESE MUSHROOMS
PULSES (LENTILS, CHICK PEAS, KIDNEY BEANS)
BROWN RICE
RED WINE, GREEN TEA
VITAMIN & MINERAL SUPPLEMENTS
ORGANIC FOOD
CLEAN WATER
FRESH AIR
EXERCISE
WEIGHT CONTROL

PART III

THE FIVE ROOTS OF GOOD HEALTH

INTRODUCTION

"We are confronted by insurmountable opportunities."

(Pogo)

This section represents the five roots of the tree: Nourishing natural foods, clean water and air, exercise and weight control, the five crucial elements to health. Ignore any one of them at your peril.

However, people do. I never cease to be amazed by people who spend fortunes on organic food, or who pour vitamin supplements down their throats whilst being 10 kilos overweight. People who pride themselves in drinking filtered water and yet have taken no exercise in years.

All five elements are equally necessary if you want to live a long and healthy life. The opportunities to eat and drink healthily, to use a gym, to take exercise, to eat in a fulfilling yet slimming way are endless. Take advantage of them.

CHAPTER 11

ORGANIC FOOD AND QUALITY, LIVING FOOD

Organic or not?

Again there is much mythology, false claim and counter claim about organic food.

What really is organic food? My definition would be that it is a natural food, grown in its fully natural state, in balance with its natural environment.

But when we cross-bred two potatoes in the eighteenth century, was the resultant potato natural? Or two breeds of chicken crossed to make a better egg-layer? Or seedless grapes, are they natural?

Now we 'play' with the natural DNA freely. The French, for example, have resisted American companies' suggestions to grow genetically modified crops. And quite right too. As we said in the introduction, our DNA evolved to be in balance with the world around it over hundreds of thousands of years. If the world around it and our foods are suddenly genetically altered, it could take hundreds of years before imbalances start to show up. That is the process of evolution, not a quick two-year crop trial.

And how can a judge decide that it is 'safe' to have a GM crop 60 yards or 80 yards from a natural one? Birds eat seeds, they fly, they deposit the seeds miles away and the next year the pollen, interacts with a natural crop. Is our evolution really to be left to ageing judges with no knowledge of science and Darwinian principles?

One estimate I read stated that there could be no natural crops in the USA in five years time. Is that what we want in Europe? For your interest I have included an **icon** article on GM foods in the Appendix.

Vitamin content

The other debate seems to centre around vitamin content. Critics of organic food say that the vegetables contain no more vitamins and minerals than mass-produced ones. And why should they?

The soils are equally depleted, even if stringent crop rotation and natural fertilisers are used.

Vitamin levels are all about the ripening process of the vegetable or fruit. If locally grown, levels should be the same for both. There are studies that suggest organic produce has more vitamins than non-organic, but there are also studies that suggest it doesn't.

What I do have is Kirlian photographs showing clearly that organic food has more 'energy' in it than non-organic. Take out of this what you will!

Pesticides and herbicides

The true benefit of organic foods is that they contact no pesticides or herbicides; no toxins to weaken our immune systems or damage the balance of hormones inside our bodies. With 'normal' vegetables and fruit there is little legislation restricting what pesticides and insecticides are used, nor how often. Over 400 fertilisers, herbicides and pesticides are available for use on our farms. Is it any wonder that farmers have a higher incidence of multiple myeloma and leukaemia?

Pesticides and insecticides have also been linked with brain tumours, connective tissue tumours (especially with children), and liver cancer and are thought to be behind the recent rapid growth of kidney cancer. Whilst individual pesticides might be found in any food at a level lower than the government's designated safe level, the government has done little research on the interaction of all the chemicals, or indeed the cumulative and interactive build up over a number of years within the tissues of the human body.

In the USA, the lifetime maximum limit set for these chemicals is exceeded when a baby reaches the age of 18 months and some of these chemicals are very hard to eliminate from our tissues once they are present.

Worse, for example, when Western governments banned DDT, they only banned its use. Some unscrupulous companies are still free to sell these dangerous chemicals to third world buyers. And do you know where your green beans and lettuce were actually grown?

Fruit orchards can be sprayed a dozen times, then the fruit is waxed locking the pesticide in. Long gone are the days when chickens populated orchards to eat the bugs, before the bugs could climb the trees!

Interestingly, not all contaminated foods were created equal! According to the Environmental Working Group of Washington DC, people can lower their pesticide exposure by 90 per cent by choosing their fruits and vegetables wisely. Eating the 12 most contaminated fruits and vegetables will expose a person to nearly 20 pesticides each day, says the EWG. In all they have now completed three studies and the findings have been consistent, with fruits worse than vegetables.

12 most contaminated		*12 least contaminated*	
Apples	Peaches	Asparagus	Mangoes
Red bell peppers	Pears	Avocados	Onions
Celery	Potatoes	Bananas	Papaya
Cherries	Red Raspberries	Broccoli	Pineapples
Grapes	Spinach	Cauliflower	Peas
Nectarines	Strawberries	Kiwi	Sweetcorn

Although this is uniquely American research it serves as an indication for all of use; we can circumvent high pesticide levels by choice. However to follow the above plan is to cut out essential ‘red’ foods from the diet. Perhaps those are best bought in ‘organic’ form if you can afford them and guarantee their authenticity.

Eat freshly picked, in season!

The Mediterranean diet is often held up as a ‘healthy’ diet, and it is very true that there are elements in it which can, and do actively prevent ill health and cancer. But what few people appreciate is how much of the food is ‘home grown’. Sixty years ago the British were urged to ‘dig for victory’. My grandfather supported his nine children from his own two allotments. Does anybody in the UK under the age of forty even grow their own vegetables now?

In contrast go and stay in any French village for a couple of weeks. Forty years ago, when the British population was 65 per cent urban, the French were still 70 per cent rural. Every village still has its large weekly market with stalls full of vegetables and fruit. The local homeowners near my house in the Var all take great pride in their often large vegetable 'patches', their fruit trees and their home grown olive and nut oils.

French TV carried a government-endorsed programme in March 2003 showing how poorer, rural and small local farmers with their limited diets of home-grown fresh vegetables and fruit had half the rates of cancer of the rest of the population.

The current estimate is that 18 per cent of French vegetables and fruits are organic, 12 per cent in Germany, 2 per cent in UK. Urbanisation kills the urge to grow things in just a generation or two.

In the Var everything has its season. In Spring we have the artichokes, then the asparagus. By late May it's the strawberries from Frejus. Then an abundance of salads, tomatoes and peppers. By August and September we are inundated with peaches, then it is figs, before the nut and mushroom festivals start in October. All grown locally, all picked and reaching you fresh. You can find your supplier and know that pesticides were not used.

In a culture which produces more and more mass farming, there is still the 'old way'. Fields near me have clearly rotated their crops each year from sunflowers, to broccoli, to grain to root vegetables. Chickens run freely in orchards to gobble up the bugs that can damage the apples. Even in Frejus, the hunters meet on Sunday mornings and the fishermen still bring their catch into the port at seven o'clock every morning. The Mediterranean people have a culture which revolves around good healthy food. Food is to be savoured, appreciated and the two-hour lunch break is still common. These principles have much in common with those developed, as we saw, in the macrobiotic diet of Japan.

The alternative is a world of large supermarket chains bringing you 'fresh' produce from all over the world, whilst increasing their volumes of higher priced organic food. (In one London supermarket I saw 'fresh organic smoked salmon, farmed in the Hebrides'!)

Why? Not because of increased consumer demand as they like to say, but because the profit margins on organic foods are higher, in a business which is having its overall margins squeezed by price wars.

Bananas are now picked completely green, packed in nitrogen-filled inert environments and shipped to you across the oceans, then via a lorry to Covent Garden, or the central supermarket warehouse. They may need 'ripening-up' a little. Strawberries from South Africa, lychees from China, mangoes from Thailand or avocados from South America. We have to be wary of 'fresh' claims for produce shipped halfway around the world. In fact you are eating unripe, rotting fruit.

Why is freshness so important? Because fruits and vegetables absorb most of their minerals and build most of their vitamins in the last throws of the ripening process. If they are picked unripe, they are picked with much lower vitamin and mineral levels. Furthermore the shipping and storing of vegetables depletes both.

Within four or five days of picking, most green vegetables have lost 50 per cent of their vitamins and a potato has lost three quarters of its vitamin C (and potatoes are the UK's best natural home-grown source of the vitamin). By the time the produce has reached the UK, then been unloaded, shipped to a central storage location and then out to the supermarkets, what nourishment can we expect to have left?

Frozen vegetables fare little better with 25 to 50 per cent of the vitamins disappearing upon freezing.

With the increasing 'faddism' in our food, which means we buy mangoes not apples, and Chinese pak-choi not British broccoli, we have to recognise that, Kirlian photography shows exactly that. Local, fresh produce has clear and strong energetic auras, imported 'old' fruit far, far less! As trendy as it seems, we are eating 'dead food'.

Unnatural and contaminated?

Of course many chemicals are added after food preparation. Nitrates and nitrites are added to make the meat look a better colour, or preserve the dried meats for longer.

Nearly 60 per cent of our processed animal products (for example meats, dairy, cheese, etc.) are fat. This fat contains toxic chemicals and antibiotics from the original animal. Over one hundred such substances have been identified and 40 per cent of them are carcinogenic[2].

Hormones, drugs and farming

In the USA 82 drugs, hormones and chemicals are allowed to be given to dairy herds. Growth hormone and oestrogen are two of these and one has to accept that any meat consumption comes with these chemicals contained in the flesh and especially the fat. Dairy consumption brings a similar chemical concoction.

Farmed meat is subject to hormone injections or antibiotics, colourings and, depending upon sources, they can have high levels of pesticides and insecticides from the fields. Farmed fish often do not consume the sorts of food they would have eaten in their natural habitat. Plankton is essential for their omega 3 levels. Farmed fish also have 20 per cent more 'fat' than their wild ancestors due to their own 'sedentary' existence!

The incidence of liver fluke in British livestock has increased four-fold since 1997 and parasites are know to weaken the human body, its immune system and cause cancer.

Viruses are another concern. BSE was brought about by feeding animal food products to herbivores. Seventeen cancers are already known to be caused by viruses. But modern farming with its focus on antibiotics, growth hormones, pesticides and high unnatural protein diets is likely to weaken the animal's immune systems laying them open to more plagues and viruses. Recently Thai prawns and chickens, which had been banned for consumption by humans because of toxins, were found to have been shipped for use by EU farmers as animal food! The toxins entered the food chain nevertheless! Animal husbandry is a fast-disappearing concept, and volume and profit margins have become the Holy Grails.

In summary

- Eat to beat cancer ideally means that you should take more trouble over selecting the products that go into your mouth. Know a few reliable suppliers. And buy locally-grown, fresh and in season. Shop more often if necessary.
- Why not start your own vegetable garden and plant fruit trees? You will be surprised how easy they are to grow along the fence instead of those leylandii.

CHAPTER 12
CLEAN WATER – THE ONLY SOLUTION

If a plant in your garden fails to grow properly, you may add nutrients to the soil and you will certainly add water. If the water is contaminated you know the plant will be affected. Why do you not use this thinking with your own health?

Clean water is essential to our health; we are, after all, 80 per cent water. It affects all our cells, our enzymatic processes and our ability to detox, and treatments such as the Gerson Therapy stress the use of pure water for cancer patients.

We suspect our tap water is polluted, but individual pollutants are below government determined safe levels. So that's all right then! And the whole issue on water safety ends up in a dispute between logic and statistics. Governments may feel there is little evidence that individual pollutants may be causing problems. But it seems logical that the combined effects may be far worse.

Rain falling brings with it smoke, dust, chemical fumes, germs, lead and strontium 90 to name but a few things. The Swedes blame the UK industrial revolution for clouds of acid rain that wiped out the fish population in some of their lakes.

Water then flows through the soil, in rivers and streams picking up fertilisers and pesticides, herbicides and nitrates.

Yummy!

Some people buy organic food only then to cook it in contaminated water; or they make their decaffeinated herb tea with boiled tap water. Boiling merely concentrates certain contaminants.

Dr Batmanghelidj, in his excellent book *Your Body's Many Cries for Water*, provides a very strong case for drinking at least two litres of water a day. Dr Batmanghelidj, trained originally at St Mary's Hospital Medical School (part of Imperial College, London). He details the research that demonstrates very convincingly that dehydration can be responsible for a huge range of ailments and degenerative diseases including dyspeptic pain, rheumatoid arthritis pain, stress and depression, high blood pressure, high blood cholesterol, excess body weight, asthma and allergies. He shows how these diseases and ailments often originate from metabolic stress, and one of the biggest contributory factors to this stress is dehydration.

In the author's postscript, Dr Batmanghelidj points out how the medical establishment are fixated on treating disease with drugs and that the pharmaceutical industry has little incentive to cure disease. He adds 'when will all NHS doctors start looking at dehydration and getting their patients to increase their clean water consumption?'

Others will argue that two litres of water per day per adult is an absolute minimum for proper cellular hydration. Three litres is probably closer to the mark and more than this might be necessary if we exercise or are sick.

If you have cancer, it is crucial to try to establish what caused the cancer so you can make every attempt to cut it out of your life. What if that toxin were water-borne?

In an Iowa study (Lynch, Zhang, Olsen) there were significantly higher levels of female lung cancer and male bladder cancer in towns with surface water supply and shadow wells. In a Finnish study on surface water (*AMJ* August 1999) chlorinated water was linked to increased incidences of bladder, kidney and stomach cancers.

Chlorine is added to water, for example, to kill germs and bacteria. Yet combined with other organic chemicals it can produce toxic chloroform. It destroys vitamin E and kills the 'friendly bacteria' in the intestinal tract. Chlorine can damage arteries and can even oxidise other contaminants in the water to produce free radicals or, worse, combine to produce chloramines which are carcinogenic. The US Environmental Agency has stated that prolonged and frequent swimming in chlorinated pools contributes to skin cancer (*Epidemiology* 1992: 3). Chlorinated water also contributes to miscarriages (*JAWWA* 1992: 20) and gastrointestinal cancer, bladder cancer and rectal cancer (*American Journal of Public Health* 1997: 87).

Several USA studies[3,4] have pointed to the links between high levels of haloforms (from chlorine) and higher levels of cancer.

Some 1000 cities now treat their water with ozone, which has had a significant effect on purity.

The *National Cancer Journal* in America has said that its study on 40 years of fluoridation showed no link to cancer. Yet in all the early tests fluorine was the tooth and bone protecting agent, and calcium fluoride the proposed additive. Now in the UK we use sodium fluoride, formerly used as a rat poison and a by-product of the aluminium industry. This water treatment is illegal in Sweden, Denmark and Holland, since apparently it can inhibit thyroid function and damage the immune system.

Furthermore, aluminium is present in significant quantities, as it is added to clarify the water during treatment. A detailed review paper[5] published in March 2002 discussed the powerful evidence showing that aluminium from drinking water and other sources is a major contributory factor to Alzheimer's disease, which is becoming increasingly common amongst older people.

Adding insult to injury, research shows that aluminium can react with low-doses of fluoride in water, causing more aluminium to cross the blood-brain barrier and become deposited in the brain. Julie Varner and her colleagues showed this definitively in a detailed 52-week study of rats, published in the prestigious peer-reviewed journal *Brain Research*[6]. Aluminium is a potent neurotoxin, and has also been implicated as a co-factor in the initiation of cancer.

Old pipes in the water system and chemicals deposited in streams can lead to lead, mercury and copper contamination. Mercury's negatives are well chronicled; both lead and copper inhibit zinc uptake in the body and zinc is important in a variety of ways from enhancing vitamin C effectiveness to protecting against prostate cancers. One theory of prostate cancer is that low levels of zinc are linked to nickel replacement.

According to scientific studies, parasites are now common in 20 per cent of the British population. In Carolina 82 per cent of the population were getting theirs from the water system as the microscopic parasites had become immune to chlorine.

A study of 22,000 women in Iowa showed that nitrate, common in rural areas was associated with bladder cancer. 20 per cent of ingested nitrate was shown to be transformed in the body to nitrite and N-nitroso compounds causing cancers such as colon and bladder (May 2001 study).

The National Academy of Sciences (September 2001) showed that even very low levels of arsenic in the water were linked to cancer (the United States EPA set standards in 1975 and may well have them wrong was the conclusion). Studies have been made from China to Chile and arsenic is increasingly found to seep into the soil from natural sources, agriculture and industrial waste.

The National Association of Scientists in America in 1998 showed that radon in the water supply was linked to lung cancers.

The latest debate concerns oestrogen levels in recycled drinking water, originating from HRT and contraceptive pills. This has been blamed for reduced fertility, and for increases in testicular cancer. Sperm count is down 20 per cent in the UK in 25 years, whilst testicular cancer is up 80 per cent. It has also been blamed for male fish showing female organ development and young human male offspring developing testicle problems and even reducing penis size.

The counter claim is that in Denmark and Scotland where there is no use of recycled water, levels are also rising. The blame is put on other chemicals in the environment, particularly endocrine disrupters like oestrogen mimics, from canned or plastic wrapped food, petrol fumes, plastics, toiletries and detergents, as we covered in Chapter 7.

Roger Lilley of Friends of the Earth blames a lack of monitoring by water companies, particularly on local rivers. Both the river Aire in Scotland and the river Lee (from where London gets drinking water) are, in varying degrees, already toxic to wildlife, according to Friends of the Earth.

Still to come is a debate about our increased consumption of drugs from statins and antibiotics to more 'exotic' chemicals. How are they taken out of recycled water?

Take action

What are we to do? Bottled water is felt to be less than perfect because of chemicals, which act as endocrine disrupters, possibly leaching from the plastic into the water in minute quantities and are carcinogenic. Boiling the water merely increases the concentration of the toxins dissolved. Distillation, if you had the time and the apparatus, can work, but it is hard to provide enough volume for all your rinsing and cooking needs on top of drinking water levels.

The best way of removing contaminants is either distillation or filtration. For an explanation of various key methods see the Appendix. Probably the simplest and best method is to use a **reverse osmosis water filter.**

One of the great advantages of this system is that you eliminate nearly all of the fluoride, parasites and bacteria, oestrogen, chlorine and aluminium in your drinking water, as well as a host of other potentially toxic chemicals so common in tap water, as long as you change the filters regularly. If you just measure the more common impurities (in parts per million), a recent test I witnessed showed scores of:

Tap water	400–700
Jug filtered tap water	275
Plastic bottled mineral water	175
Reverse osmosis filtered	6

Whether you already have cancer or are keen to prevent it, you should take a realistic view of the above facts and take action.

Water is vital to your body and health.

Keep it clean.

CHAPTER 13

FRESH AIR – THE ENEMY OF CANCER

If a blood sample of a cancer sufferer is placed under a microscope two things are usually observed. Firstly, the white, immune system cells are 'lifeless' whereas in normal blood they move around. Secondly, the red cells are often clumped together – a sign that both iron and oxygen-carrying levels are low.

Cancer cells resemble very primitive cell forms as we discussed earlier. Whereas normal cells burn carbohydrate in oxygen to produce their energy, cancer cells do not use oxygen, and their waste product is lactic acid, the toxic substance more usually associated with cramp. This lactic acid is very hard to break down and further pollutes the localised environment. It has to be oxygenated by the liver to clear it from the body.

The fact that cancer cells are anaerobic or partially anaerobic 'organisms' and they do not need oxygen to thrive means they actually prefer a medium with little oxygen. Moreover oxygen can actually kill cancer cells.

In 1931, Otto Warburg won a Nobel Prize for this discovery. Since then, German and American scientists have pioneered treatments which aim to get oxygen into cancer cells. Hence the 'alternative' therapies, which use high doses of vitamin C, ozone or hydrogen peroxide as pre-oxidants to get inside the cell and 'oxidise' it.

Warburg himself concluded that the best way to fight cancer was to get oxygen to the cancer cells and to do this you needed oxygenated arteries (as is normally the case) and oxygenated veins (normally very low in oxygen) to create a 'bottleneck' and a cellular overload. Since veins carry about 70 per cent of the body's blood volume with about 13 per cent inside the organs, this is a difficult feat to achieve, but the theory of blood oxygen overload has taxed some of the world's best cancer specialists for the last 70 years.

Certain factors work against blood oxygen levels. As we have said elsewhere, high levels of oestrogen depress cellular oxygen; depression itself limits blood oxygen.

For all of us, it is absolutely imperative we keep our bloodstreams well oxygenated. There are a number of ways to do this. Moderate exercise will build your oxygen carrying capacity and it is vital that we each take at least 30 minutes of exercise daily, coupled with deep breathing. It is quite worrying that in a UK report in February 2003, 20 per cent of school children did not do any weekly exercise.

Deep breathing exercises are part of the Chinese programme for cancer sufferers and the fact is that most of us do not breathe properly. Unless we do something strenuous we tend only to use the top third of our lung capacities, allowing toxic air to sit and stagnate at the bottom of our lungs. This prevents toxins moving out of our bloodstreams and into our lungs to be excreted.

Correct iron levels will help too and many foods, especially green vegetables, are excellent sources of readily assimilated organic iron. Excess dairy consumption can restrict iron levels.

But the world is against us. Thc biggest direct hazard to our blood oxygen is smoking, with its carbon monoxide level, which blocks the haemoglobin oxygen carrying sites; passive smokers have been shown to be six times more threatened than was originally thought and women are twice as prone to the damaging effects of smoke as negative airway factors have been found to be carried by the X chromosome – women have two X chromosomes, men just one (Cancer Research UK).

The air we breathe makes us vulnerable to a host of diseases including cancer. Motor vehicles emit hazardous toxic chemicals, which collect on dust and, especially under the effect of sunlight, become toxic particles. These collect in the deepest recesses of your lungs and are virtually impossible to clear out. This results in increased levels of toxins in the bloodstream, with further toxins collecting in body fat and organs like the kidneys. Diesel fumes have been decreed as the third largest cause of lung cancer in the USA.

Polluted cities can have oxygen levels as low as 12 per cent on a bad day compared with the 21 per cent of air normally attributed to oxygen. At 7 per cent life ceases.

General air pollution is also hazardous to human life. The US Environmental Agency reports that over a hundred million tonnes of various toxic chemicals are released into the atmosphere every year in the USA. *The Nation* (September 17 1990) reported that autopsies on one hundred young people in the Los Angeles region showed that all had lungs suffering from toxic air pollution damage.

In summary

If you want to prevent cancer, and certainly if you have it already, it is crucial you give serious consideration to where you live, and how to get a good source of quality oxygen into your lungs on a regular basis.

- Do not smoke, do not have people in your home who smoke.
- Do not live near main roads or sources of diesel fumes.
- Live well away from factories or other sources of air pollution.
- Learn to use your lungs and breathe properly.
- Take . . . exercise.

CHAPTER 14

EXERCISE – ARE YOU FIT ENOUGH TO BEAT CANCER?

Medical science has proven conclusively that fit people are ill less. And fit people recover quicker after an illness or an operation.

Researchers at the University of Bristol have conducted an extensive review of 52 international studies on exercise and found that physical activity can significantly reduce the risk of bowel cancer and may help prevent breast, prostate, lung and endometrial cancer. They found compelling evidence on bowel cancer that regular exercise could cut the risk of developing the disease by 40–50 per cent.

From 37 of the 52 studies on exercise and breast cancer incidence, scientists found evidence that showed typically a 30 per cent reduction in the risk of the disease in women who exercised on a regular basis. Generally, the benefits of exercise were stronger for post-menopausal women than pre-menopausal women.

Other studies have shown that cancers of the colon, lung, kidney and rectum have all been linked to a sedentary lifestyle, a lack of exercise and surplus weight.

Finnish researchers have examined exercise in the general context of cancer and shown that poor fitness increases your odds of cancer statistically in line with, say, smoking. In fact, they further concluded, that exercise also helps fight cancer. The Bristol researchers also produced data showing that exercise can help patients better recover from cancer.

Interestingly in 2003 researchers at Fred Hutchinson Cancer Research Center, Seattle, showed that exercise did not have to be strenuous. Women who exercised a little, but every day, reduced their risk of breast cancer 17 per cent.

The Center for Integrative Medicine, Thomas Jefferson University Hospital, Philadelphia, studied cortisol levels amongst over 10,000 people.

Typically in stressed situations, the brain stimulates the adrenals to produce cortisol. A doctor might tell you to go home and rest. Researchers found resting would reduce cortisol levels just 5 per cent, whereas your first ever yoga class reduced levels nearly 25 per cent.

What is 'being fit'?

A lot is written about the Chinese and their low rates of cancer, but usually only in the context of diet. To attempt to cross the street in a rural town in China is risking death by a thousand bicycles. Chinese people walk, pull carts and cycle well into their old age. 60 million alone practice Tai Chi daily!

Meanwhile most British people 'kid' themselves they are fit. "I'm fit, I walk the dog most days." "I'm fit, I have a regular game of golf every Sunday." "I'm fit, I do the gardening." Our lives are basically sedentary; office work, watching TV, driving the car. A game of golf once a week does not make you fit, even if it is on a highly undulating course.

The government doesn't help. It puts out official statements like 'to be fit you should do twenty minutes aerobic exercise, three times per week.' It doesn't sound much does it? An hour of walking the dog must surely qualify. It doesn't.

A study by MORI in January 2003 showed that less than 20 per cent of women even did that much exercise. Or should I say, that little!

The Government Health Authority's official recommendation is that during this twenty minutes you should exercise consistently and constantly with a certain and quite high heart rate. Before that you should gradually warm up, and afterwards gradually cool down adding a further ten minutes either side. So it's really 40 minutes.

During the middle 20 minutes you should be working throughout at 85 per cent of your maximum heart rate. This is calculated as follows. Take your age away from 220, and then take 85 per cent of it. For a man of 60 the work out should consist of twenty minutes where you heart rate is consistently at around 136 beats per minute (220 – 60 = 160 x 85% = 136).

Could you do that? Walking the dog will see your heart rate reach around 95 beats per minute if you amble along. A four hour round of golf may see you peak at 120 a couple of times for 30 seconds or so if the course is hilly.

What really is fitness? Surely it is a combination of a number of things, for example:

- Normal, not high, blood pressure
- Flexibility
- Muscular strength
- Heart power and stamina

Diet will help your blood pressure, but so too will being fit. Stretching and yoga will help the flexibility, whilst weights and cycling, power walking, running and swimming will help the last two.

Right now in the UK, gyms, health clubs and sports centres are booming and the growth area comes from the 28–35 age group and particularly the 50 plus age group. So there's no excuse. Buy the tracksuit and trainers and join your peers at the health centre! Eight to twelve weeks of three times per week will see a difference starting to take place. And you never know, you might even enjoy it.

But you will have to work at it. If you are out of shape now you have a greater risk of disease and you cannot expect to correct years of ignoring your body in one or two weeks. You need to make a lifetime commitment. Surely your life is worth a little daily effort, isn't it? You are proud of the clothes you wear and your achievements. Why not be proud of your body and your health?

The basic rule with fitness is to 'think active' – try to be active every day. Don't leave it to the official three days a week. In one study, a natural sample of everyday Chinese were burning 3500 calories per week in exercise. That's the equivalent of one hour on the bike in the gym every day! By all means go to the health club for professional advice, but on your days off, speed walk with the dog, take a cycle ride, go for a swim and try to do something every day. It will pay dividends.

Build muscle, lose toxins

Too many people set unrealistic goals of weight loss in short periods of time for their new-found exercise routines. Don't. One pound of fat contains approximately 3000 calories so at the outset you will not lose it quickly, especially when you consider that your first hour on the bicycle in the gym will burn around 400 calories. You need to get several things working hard for you and that takes some time.

But even the longest road starts with the first step. You start to burn fat after roughly 12 minutes of aerobic exercise, and fat stores toxins in your body because it is a very good solvent. Immediately you start to lose fat, you will start to lose some of the stored toxins.

And over the weeks as you rebuild some lost muscle, an upward spiral starts. For every pound of muscle you add to your body, you burn 30 calories per day just to maintain it. So by losing three pounds of fat and gaining three pounds of muscle you might feel gloomy when you stand on the scales, but over a week the extra muscle will be burning a 1000 calories or so, even when you have a day off and are sitting watching the TV. Given the daily recommended intake for a woman of 1500–1800 calories and a man at 2200–2800 calories you can see that the benefits will start to grow. Stick at it. Bear in mind that we are not talking about building 'muscles', just converting some of the fat back into the state it was, in your youth.

As you work out over the weeks you will find your programme easier. Increases in muscle result in increased levels of creatine kinase, an important muscle and energy enzyme, which will help burn calories and make all your activities seem easier to perform.

Drink plenty of water after your exercise to flush out those toxins, and eat protein within two hours of the work out to rebuild the muscle.

Release the hormones

Working out produces endorphins, often called happy hormones. Not only will they fight depression, they will neutralise the stress hormones in your body. Stress hormones have a negative effect on your cellular environment by stimulating the production of bad eicosanoids, as we discussed in Chapter 8. Active exercise helps the biochemical environment of every cell in your body. It's illogical to spend lots of money on antioxidants and toxin-free products if at the same time you allow your cells to float in stressed, toxic surroundings.

Lifting weights to a point of having tired muscles, will also cause Human Growth Hormone (Hgh) to be produced. If you are over 50 years of age you are hardly making this hormone any more. Along with melatonin, it is produced about one and a half hours into your sleep when young. But resistance training will produce a shot of growth hormone at almost any age.

Hgh is a powerful neutraliser of free radicals, and helps to further eliminate fatty deposits and builds lean muscle. In research studies in America with Hgh, people over 50 reported regaining lean muscle mass, losing fat and feeling youthful and re-vitalised. Go to the gym and ask the instructors to help you with resistance training. It helps men and women avoid osteoporosis too, without the need for supplements like HRT. You will gradually feel lighter, happier and re-energised as the months pass.

Oxygenate your cells

Most fitness books talk about the benefits to your heart and circulatory systems and it is true that you should see a gradual improvement in your blood pressure and your peripheral cardio-vascular system. Your heart will become stronger and your blood more oxygenated.

Your lungs will learn to work again. As we said in the last chapter, most people who take no exercise only use a third of their lung capacity, the other two thirds has stagnant, polluted and toxic air sitting in it. The blood passing in the tissues next to this air cannot get rid of its toxins in to that polluted air. When working out aerobically you will fill your lungs and expel this dead air. This will help clear out the toxins and get more oxygen into your bloodstream. And oxygen is the enemy of cancer cells as we covered before.

As the blood system strengthens it will carry this oxygen to the most distant cells much more efficiently than before.

Move your lymph

Meanwhile your cells are bathed in a fluid called lymph. You have twice as much lymph in your body as you have blood. The only problem is that the lymph system has no heart to pump it round the body. When you sleep at night, your whole lymph system 'sleeps'. What will you do to wake it up?

The largest lymph duct is the thoracic duct, which passes across your chest. You must move your lymph daily to clear toxins away from your cells. And you must replace it with clean lymph, which is where exercise and clean water enter the equation.

Aerobic exercise pumps your heart faster and this stimulates the thoracic duct. Certain exercises, like breaststroke swimming, press-ups and yoga also get the chest moving. Even yawning and laughing help move the lymph across the chest.

Exercise will improve your posture, which in turn helps remove restrictions on your lymph and energy flow.

As your peripheral circulation improves, so too will your peripheral lymph system allowing the toxins to move out of even the most distant cells. Stretching, like massage can help with this lymphatic drainage.

Exercise – the best detox?

So, the environment around your cells is cleaner, more oxygen is being supplied to your tissues and nutrients are being more efficiently transported. More muscle raises the metabolic rate of the whole body encouraging it to work more efficiently and to control the levels of fat. As the toxins move away in the lymph, they pass into the bloodstream and are expelled through the lungs, or in the urine, or through the liver. Human growth hormone and endorphins help to de-fat the liver and stimulate its action. Even a simple sit-up will stimulate your intestines into action aiding the expulsion of the toxins from the bile ducts and the intestines.

No need for 'the burn'

If you find all this sensible, but are daunted by images of lycra-clad lovelies 'going for the burn', be reassured. Too much exercise produces even more toxins in the body, burns up certain vitamins and is probably counter productive. This is part of the reason why so many top athletes are so often ill or end up with diabetes. Exercise for health should simply be a sensible, controlled and long-term commitment to a healthier you. "*Never confuse motion with action*", as Ernest Hemingway said. You may see much motion down the gym but the best regimes are planned action programmes for health not slimming.

Take the first step

Cancer Research UK and Tesco published research in February 2003 which showed that one in four women take no exercise at all, whilst the majority of women do less than the government recommended minimum. One in five women were honest enough to admit they simply lacked the motivation!

In summary

- Realise this is a commitment for life, not a quick three-week fix.
- To repeat: **Don't measure your gain in fitness by weight loss**.
- You may even put weight on at first because muscle is heavier than fat. But if you 'think active' and exercise regularly over a six-month period you will change shape and lose weight. By all means couple the exercise programme with a diet and some lifestyle changes.
- Be disciplined. Take professional advice and follow it. Ask for a specific programme that's right for your age; too many gyms give the same programme to an 18-year-old and a 58-year-old. Allow one and a half hours, an hour to work out and thirty minutes of showering and changing. Take the time for yourself. You are worth it.
- Find a friend to go with you, make a date to see him or her at a regular time on certain days. Stick at it.
- Set yourself goals, but not the sort that read, "I want to lose 10 pounds in 10 weeks". They are incredibly meaningless and unattainable. Set a goal for this year. Ask the health club to measure your fat content and set a target goal for fat. Or, "in six months time I'm going to be able to ride a bike for

thirty minutes at 80 revolutions per minute". These are goals that deliver health.

- And above all enjoy yourself. Meet new people and have new vitality. You've only got one life – so make the most of it.

CHAPTER 15

WEIGHT CONTROL – TAKING PRIDE IN YOURSELF

We have all read reports that being overweight is bad for your health. And, let's be honest, most of us ignore them. Well consider this: Erasmus College Rotterdam reanalysed American population data taken over a fifty-year period and concluded if you were forty years old and just four kilograms overweight you reduced your life expectancy by 3 years. At ten or more kilograms the loss was 7 years for women and 5.6 for men. Furthermore, overweight people pay 12 per cent more visits to the doctor each year and spend 19 per cent longer per year in hospital (Men's Health UK, 2002).

And try this for size: **People who are overweight get more cancer**. Fact.

The Organisation for Economic Co-operation and Development published a report in October 2002 stating that the UK has the second highest level of obesity in the world after the USA. With 21 per cent obesity we follow the USA at 26 per cent. By contrast the Swiss are Europe's best at 6.8 per cent and the Japanese have a lowly 2.9 per cent. The UK Under Secretary for Health, Hazel Blears, said, "*There are clear links between obesity and our biggest killers, heart disease and cancer.*"

Everyday you burn energy inside your cells. The more energy you burn, the more waste products you produce; and the more waste products, the more your cells are toxic. Eat more and you have more toxic cells.

People who are overweight tend to be less active. As mentioned in the previous chapter, one of your body's natural defences is its lymph system. But the lymph needs to be flowing past your cells to take the toxins away. Overweight people and older people tend to be more sedentary reducing lymph flow. So their cells are more toxic.

Overweight people are often thus because of poor eating habits and a poor diet. Poor quality eating habits form at an early age.

One third of UK boys under six are overweight or obese, rising to almost 50 per cent by the age of 16. In the USA it is 60 per cent.

47 per cent of children eat no vegetables other than potato in a month and a recent survey showed that half of ten-year-olds could not even recognise certain vegetables like broccoli correctly.

People who eat badly (more fatty foods, sugary foods, salt processed and preserved foods, fried foods, etc) are putting more free radicals into their bodies. So their cells are more toxic.

Overweight people have more stores of fat in their bodies. Firstly, it is now known that for both men and women excess fat can produce oestrogen in the body. Also fat, as we've said repeatedly, is a wonderful solvent. So more toxins are dissolved by the fat and held in the body. Fat people have more, 'toxic cells'. Think of it as toxic waist!

Overweight people often have hormone imbalances because of extra amounts of hormones trapped in their fat and the hormones stored within it can even reach near dangerous levels. Drinking several cans of fizzy soft drink, or eating a high starch/carbohydrate meal simply stresses the imbalances by increasing insulin levels causing the body's hormones to be thrown out of balance even more.

In laboratory tests, the rats that consumed 10 per cent less calories than they needed, lost their excess fat stores over time, storing and holding less hormones and toxins. Less ingested calories also meant less burnt calories and less waste, and a better control of hormone production. Their metabolism and biochemistry was more regular, more controlled and they were less toxic. They lived to the human equivalent of 140 years of age.

As we saw in Chapter 8, eating more fats just increases the fatty acid pool in the body. This in turn increases the potential for harmful eicosanoids around the cells, unless you are eating a lot of fish and omega 3 or ginger and garlic, which can all turn off the controlling enzymes. So, again overweight people have more toxic cells.

If overweight people can break the cycle and lose some excess weight they will naturally feel better and become more active.

Many psychologists will tell you that excessive smoking, drinking or eating stems from emotional problems. One of the biggest hurdles to overcome for the would-be slimmer is to actually respect themselves. "I am important, my family loves me, I have good friends, I like living, I am fun, and I have worth and value." If you respect yourself, you value yourself. And if you value someone or something, you want to spend time on them and appreciate them. So appreciate yourself. Start to respect your body, lose a little weight and eat better.

The first hurdle is the first couple of kilos. If you can kick start a slimming programme, you will feel happier and more self motivated, and this allows you to go on to bigger things. Isn't it time you valued yourself a little more and lost those first few kilos? A mild food restriction diet that places the emphasis on low animal fat while eating organic foods, coupled with a detox, light exercise and saunas or steam baths might be a good combination to start with.

One report I read recently said that overweight people had 40 per cent more risk of getting cancer. By contrast, smoking 'only' increased the risk by 25 per cent

How about those figures for size?

In summary

- Being overweight greatly increases your risks of cancer, more so than smoking. By contrast people who are 5 per cent below ideal weight or people on restricted diets increase their longevity. Calorie and fat control is crucial. Eat less!
- Respect and love yourself. Be proud of your looks and your body. Take care of it. It needs to last you a lifetime.

PART IV

SUPPORTING ACT

INTRODUCTION

"It's not the men in my life that counts – it's the life in my men".

(Mae West)

This section is the trunk, or the support, of the tree and concerns the need to gain the maximum value from your diet in terms of vitamins and minerals.

Factors such as yeasts and parasites are working against this, weakening your essential vitamin and mineral intake and your immune system.

Supplementation is important to good health. In some instances it is essential. It is neither 'useless' nor an expensive luxury.

There is an important difference between 'living life' and 'living life in top form, in excellent health'. Some people believe they are in good health until something tests them, be it a bad cold or a mystery virus. Being in excellent health is the ability to live life in top gear; the ability of the body to meet any challenge, big or small.

CHAPTER 16

MICROBES – THE THIEVES OF NOURISHMENT

In my first book, *Everything You Need to Know to Help You Beat Cancer*, I covered yeasts, viruses and parasites extensively.

A short summary would be:

- 17 cancers are already known to be caused by viruses. As detection methods become more refined who knows how many the final total will be?
- Parasites are felt to have a link to cancer. In one study 42 out of 1000 patients in a USA cancer hospital were found to have a liver fluke; this was eradicated and many treated patients recovered. Parasites can be microscopic and come with imported fruit, become guests on a foreign holiday, can come in the water supply (microscopic parasites are becoming increasingly chlorine resistant), and fluke in British livestock has increased four-fold since 1997.
- Yeasts are thought to be present in 70 per cent of the UK population, and are often living undetected.
- Whilst viruses can 'infect' cells, and parasites can produce carcinogenic toxins into the blood supply, all three (viruses, parasites and yeasts) also have a severe draining effect on all vitamins in the body, particularly B vitamins. Several B vitamins are crucial in their cancer protection role: biotin boosts the immune system, choline and inositol help de-fat the liver and folic acid is vital for accurate DNA replication. Furthermore, the immune system will also be weakened when attempting to cope with the presence of any, or all, of these invaders.

When researching cancer I came across several eminent reports that every cancer sufferer had one of these natural invaders.

Certainly this theory seems ever more likely. For example, more and more evidence is being produced on the role of

Helicobacter pylori in stomach cancers. This bacterium 'hides' from the acid in the stomach by diving into the mucous membrane. This causes the immune system to rush to the other side of the lining, setting up the conditions for an ulcer. A similar but more complex process seems to set up a cancer too. Acidophilus is known to keep Helicobacter pylori in check, but not to eradicate it. Acid will kill the bacterium but as we age, we produce less. When you pass the age of 50, you produce 20 to 30 per cent less acid. However, the way we eat, the very fact we confuse our stomachs by eating protein and carbohydrate mixes (like pepperoni pizza, or tuna sandwiches, or seafood pasta) reduces the acid levels in our stomachs. Our stomachs produce acid in response to proteins, but alkali in response to carbohydrates. Mix the two and acidity levels fall making Helicobacter pylori a happy bacterium.

Helicobacter pylori infection is also associated with low blood levels of vitamin B-12 and folic acid, both essential in the anti-cancer process. Only recently, women with breast cancer were shown to have lowered levels of vitamin B-12. 73 per cent of vegetarians have insufficient B-12 as its main source is animal. (An algae, Chlorella, is an excellent source too.)

A tetracycline antibiotic can kill off Helicobacter pylori, and this is helped by the trace mineral bismuth – the simplest source of which is a quality colloidal mineral supplement like Neways Maximol.

Microbe, virus, bacteria and yeast detection is best done by qualified homeopaths who use analytical systems like VEGA; the homeopaths can then help you work to eradicate these unwelcome polluters. In Germany the use of such 'alternative' systems is far more commonplace than in the UK and is available on the state health service to all patients.

In the last six months I have visited a number of specialist cancer clinics. In every case, I always go and talk to the people at the 'sharp end', the nurses!

What has astounded me is that they have all been adamant that **every** cancer patient they treat has a bad yeast infection, or candida – **women and men**. Worse, back in 1993 *Contemporary Oncology*, a major cancer magazine for doctors in the USA stated clearly that people suffering from cancer who had radiotherapy and or chemotherapy did not die from these cancers “but finally succumbed to an infestation of candida albicans” (yeasts!).

Perhaps the best way of thinking of ‘yeasts’ and similar ‘infections’ is to regard them as microbes. Candida infection is an infection of microbes.

So what causes microbial infection?

As we said above, parasites can come from a variety of sources. A trend to sushi (raw fish) and lightly cooked meats also does not help.

Yeasts may be thought of a little as you would ‘fire’ – fire is helpful to humans in a controlled form, but devastating if allowed to get out of control. Gerald Green is the grandson of Professor Fritz Haber who discovered how to fix nitrogen leading to an understanding of a number of substances from fertilisers to explosives. Gerald is extremely knowledgeable about candida and I am indebted to him for increasing my knowledge.

Apparently our ‘friendly’ bacteria feed off the yeasts and amoeba at night whilst we sleep. One estimate I read said that in a healthy individual the ‘friendly’ bacteria could devour up to two pounds of these yeasts and microbes a night! But if the ‘friendly’ bugs are killed, the yeasts multiply unchecked.

The prime culprits for killing the friendly bugs are antibiotics and highly chlorinated tap water. Or steroids and chemotherapy used in orthodox cancer treatments. Even extreme acidity in the body caused by our lifestyles and diets can damage the friendly population. The friendly bugs can be wiped out in just three days in bad conditions.

This creates a ‘double whammy’.

Firstly, the ‘friendly bacteria’ are essential to your good health. They aid digestion, they are the first line of defence in the immune system (indeed, they can actually synthesise biotin, one of the immune boosting vitamins); and most importantly recent research has shown that pieces of their cell walls actually kill cancer cells *in vitro*. (This last finding is fascinating and has surprised many doctors.)

Secondly, the bacteria normally keep the yeasts in check, but with no friendly bacteria, the yeasts multiply and grow. Yeasts grow like mushrooms, in that they have 'roots' that can pass across the gut wall into the bloodstream. Toxins may then pass directly into your bloodstream and greatly weaken the immune system. This is turn causes further illness, for which more antibiotics may be prescribed. This vicious circle frequently occurs, for example, in tonsillitis. Worse, the candida microbes can leave the gut and themselves pass into the bloodstream causing all sorts of havoc.

The most devastating effect of these microbes is their role in cancer, a role that, frankly, remains completely unconsidered by the majority of the general medical profession in the UK.

Candida microbes, apart from feasting on the nutrients your immune system needs, produce an 'alcohol'. This poisons the bloodstream, making you feel 'hung over' and lethargic and invoking serious work from your liver to detoxify it. Even worse, it feeds the cancer cells. **This alcohol produces the same by-product as fat does, and cancer cells thrive on it.** There is even a view that such yeasts are anaerobes and can 'cluster' in certain areas of the body turning adjacent cells into anaerobes (i.e. cells 'working' without oxygen). Such cells are the basis of cancer.

So what can you do about yeasts?

The answer is two-fold: diet and supplement. You cannot maintain health just with diet.

For dietary control it is essential that you cut out all sugars, all alcohol, all cow's milk and all yeasts. If you continue to ingest these items, the candida microbes will thrive.

Sugar in any form (lactose, dextrose, glucose, honey etc) is loved by candida, as is very sweet fruit. Indeed several books on diets tell you only to eat fruit on an empty stomach in the morning. This would not be the case if you were yeast-free. There would be no need to follow this advice. In Thailand or China they eat fruit any time and before or after meals, but then much of their diet is anti-yeast. However, where candida microbes abound, fruit or even certain vegetables like cucumber, marrows, courgettes and squash, can sit on top of the food in the stomach and ferment.

Ingesting natural yeasts (for example, mushrooms, bread, Oxo cubes) is equally bad news. And of course over-ripe fruit and alcohol are full of both sugars and yeasts! Junk foods, fast foods, branded fruit juices, processed foods and foods from crisps to breakfast cereals often contain both yeasts and sugars. Go fresh and home cooked!

Finally cow's milk is taboo for a number of reasons. Lactose, sugar found in cow's milk, allows yeasts to thrive; dairy has many negative effects on the minerals supporting the immune system covered earlier in this book; and it is hard to digest. Where candida is associated with 'leaky gut syndrome', dairy can directly poison the blood system.

When attempting an anti-candida diet, Gerald Green recommends participants avoid too much carbohydrate, especially refined carbohydrate as this can turn to sugar. For example, he recommends avoiding:

- Bread and all relatives
- Cereals, hot or cold
- All snack products from crisps to popcorn
- All white rice, potatoes, corn and refined wheat products like pasta
- Most fruit
- Root vegetables
- Lentils, chickpeas, dried beans
- All coffee, caffeine, fizzy soft drinks, fruit juices, alcohol
- All convenience/junk foods
- All cow's dairy
- All processed meat products (bacon, sausages, salami)
- All high salt foods
- All mushrooms and fungi
- All condiments
- All hydrogenated fatty acids and saturated fats
- Health supplements containing lactose, gluten and citric acid.

His good food choices include:

- Alfalfa and sprouting seeds
- Sweet peppers

- Broccoli, brussel sprouts, cauliflower, cabbage and greens, kale, chard
- Endive, fennel, garlic, onions, spring onions
- Green beans
- Hot chilli peppers
- Lettuce, spinach
- Parsley
- Radishes
- Olive oil, flaxseed oil, fish oil
- Eight glasses of water per day
- Herb teas
- Free range eggs
- Fresh fish
- Pork, lamb, veal
- Chicken, turkey, game
- Quorn, soya milk, rice milk, sheep's and goat's milk
- Soda bread (wheat free) with no added sugar or salt.

It is interesting to note that foods like garlic and hot chilli peppers are the staples in the Far East for keeping microbial infection at bay. Fresh garlic, when you cut it, oozes like a fresh potato. It does not have a green stem in the middle, nor does it appear as concentric leaves like an onion. It doesn't smell and it is hot on the stomach. Two cloves a day uncooked would be good. (If you buy the 'leafy' variety in your supermarket, you should know that taking the green centre out avoids the stale 'garlic' smell.)

Microbes and their control is one area where supplementation is vital. For example, you may take garlic oil or cloves, oregano, slippery elm, caprylic acid (coconut) and Pau d'Arco. In fact, Pau d'Arco was thought at one point to be a cure for cancer. It comes from the bark of a South American tree and is a really excellent anti-bacterial, anti-viral, and anti-yeast agent. It is not, after all, an anti-cancer agent but its powers against factors that might cause the cancer or weaken the immune system are beyond question. Gerald Green himself recommends wormwood (Artemisia Absinthium), an anti-parasitic herb used for many years as a digestive tonic. He also recommends half a teaspoonful of freshly ground cinnamon in a glass of water. It helps fight the candida in the bloodstream, reduces sugar levels and stops the microbes forming the alcohol used by the cancer cells. (N.B. Patients with Type 1 diabetes must not use this.)

In South East Asia bee propolis and bee pollen are also used extensively.

The 'intestine war' between 'friendly bacteria' and the yeasts will almost certainly have drawn your body energy to your intestine area. It is worth visiting a cranial osteopath or acupuncturist to have your energy rebalanced throughout your body.

Homeopaths have nosodes (natural potions that stimulate disease responses) to treat yeasts and these too can be very helpful. You should, undoubtedly, take a probiotic too, like aeidophilus to top-up levels of the good guys.

And, when you undergo your 'yeast cleanse', you must also aim to restrengthen your immune system. The following would be helpful.

Vitamin C	Twice per day, 500 mgs each time
Vitamin E	400 IU
Beta-carotene	Twice per day, 6 mgs each time
Zinc	15 mgs
Selenium	200 micrograms yeast-free
B complex	1 tablet (but only a yeast-free tablet)

Echinacea and astragalus are also recommended by Green. If you have to sweeten things, use Stevia, it is a natural leaf sweetener and apart from being considerably sweeter than sugar it has anti-fungal and anti-bacterial properties. (Stevia can be obtained in the USA but is not on general sale in the UK.)

Finally, psyllium seeds should be added to the diet (2 tablespoons per day), the diet should be high in natural fibre, and at least 2 litres of water should be consumed per day (but not with meals).

In summary

- There is no doubt that microbes cause illnesses. Many residents of the Western world have yeasts and some have parasites. Keeping them in check is vital.
- Cancer sufferers could do well to go on a two–three week

'purge' especially since, as Green says, wormwood is fast acting and may only require a few days to take effect.

- People wishing to prevent cancer might treat this as a twice yearly 'cleanse', and then use the rest of the year keeping candida microbes at bay by limiting their nutritionally empty sugar, their alcohol and their dairy and yeast consumptions.
- When microbes 'drain' us of our vitamins, minerals and our very 'life force' it is essential to supplement to remove them and also to replace the life they have taken out of us.
- Everybody should think seriously about having a VEGA or BEST test to ensure they are clear of microbes (yeasts and parasites) and viruses. For cancer patients this is a 'must'.

CHAPTER 17

SUPPLEMENTS – WHAT DOCTORS CAN'T TELL YOU

As I said earlier, I am full of praise for doctors. During my quest to find out things to aid my daughter's cancer fight I came to realise that, of course, they are rarely qualified to advise on nutrition, biochemistry or body energy. They are rarely qualified to advise on supplements either. They may never cover these things during their seven years of academic qualifications.

Fair's fair. I won't give advice on chemotherapy, I promise.

Unfortunately, a number of unqualified people choose to make sweeping comments in the media about supplements, usually in a negative way. 'Vitamins are useless' was the key phrase in 2002 after Professor Rory Collins of Oxford University conducted research into statins with 20,000 heart problem patients over five years in the UK. The research was in part funded by Merck who make statins. Three antioxidants were chosen in a side-by-side test and had no effect on the survival rates of the heart patients. First, expert nutritionists could have recommended supplements more likely to succeed than the three chosen. Second, somehow the results of the research (I read the original report in *The Lancet*) were mysteriously extrapolated in the media and interpreted as "*Oxford Professor says all supplements are useless*", "*a waste of money, the money would be better spent on fresh vegetables and fruit*", and worse "*vitamins are useless even in treatment of cancer*". Where the last conclusion came from, goodness knows. It certainly wasn't in the research study. Why are we subjected to this nonsense in the media?

The nonsense doesn't stop there. The Food Standards Agency in the UK is quite clear "You don't need supplements if you eat a 'balanced diet'". So we asked them to define a balanced diet and they said that it should be built around 'starchy foods', have five lots of fruit and vegetables per day, and contain a little of everything (we have the letter!). What nonsense is this? Nowadays, starchy foods like pasta, bread, etc are largely refined – the sort of foods that give 8 per cent of adults in the USA late onset diabetes (and under-12s in the USA a staggering 16 per cent!).

A little of everything? Some oils (polyunsaturated) will destroy vitamins like beta-carotene and even a little saturated fat could build up over time depending upon the individual. Does the FSA advocate a little smoking and a little alcohol as well for the same reasons?!

But then 2003 has also seen the peak of the EU vitamin directive debate. There is a desire by those well-paid people in power to restrict the number of vitamins and mineral supplements on sale in Europe. Few people realise the extent of the restrictions. Some 300 of 420 'common' vitamins and minerals will no longer be on sale from 2005–6. Synthetic products, not natural organic ones, will be almost the only supplements available for sale on the high street, all at levels in line with recommended daily allowances (RDAs). Except that a number of crucial supplements have been left off the short-list, scientifically researched RDAs do not even exist for some supplements, and many of the decisions are transparently rather less than scientific. I suppose, worst of all, wc have recently learned that vitamins like vitamin D, which was thought to be the preventer of rickets now does far more and is a strong fighter of cancer. The last five years have seen similar advances in our knowledge of vitamin K and its role with liver cancer and leukaemia. The levels being shown in the USA to have anti-cancer benefits are greatly above the currently approved RDAs. It seems crazy to realise that just as the scientists are making breakthrough discoveries (and let's be honest, the knowledge of the biochemistry of vitamins is really still in its infancy) the government is making decisions based on 60-year-old data, some of which is now known to be limited or inapplicable.

So, it seems, we are not just under attack from our toxic environments, but from misinformed media and biased bureaucracy.

Let's just have a look at the truth:

- Our soils are increasingly depleted. Crops are grown for volume and frequency, crop rotation is rarely used, natural seasons have been shortened, resulting in certain fields barely even rested as one crop of wheat follows another.
- In February 2004 David Thomas, a minerologist, published

a paper investigating the decline of minerals in our fruits and vegetables from 1940 to 1990, using the government's own figures. It showed major declines in potassium, magnesium, iron and calcium. A second, separate study, by Anne-Marie Mayer of Cornell University was published in the *Bristol Food Journal* and made similar conclusions.

- Curiously the EU and the US governments are completely at odds. Whilst the EU seeks to minimize our intake of vitamins and minerals, the US government has long been telling us to most definitely take them. Starting with a clear statement in the Senate minutes in 1936 that laboratory tests had proven that US farm soils were becoming minerally depleted, as was the produce, and that people were developing deficiencies. Even in 2002 similar pro-supplement statements were being made by US health authorities.

But our weakened soils are only the start. Other factors reduce your vitamin and mineral intake and nourishment as we have seen. To recap:

- Much of the produce we eat has travelled a long distance. It may be a week between picking and eating, or more.
- Broccoli, brassicas, spinach, asparagus lose 50 per cent of their vitamins within five days of picking. A potato will lose 75 per cent of its vitamin C within 5 days. Fruits can lose 50 per cent of their vitamin C within 1 day.
- Much of the produce we eat, especially fruit, has been picked unripe so that it does not go off during the week or so that it takes to reach you.
- Fruits gain the majority of their vitamins as they ripen. Unripe fruit may be 50 to 60 per cent deficient.
- Even frozen vegetables lose about a third of their vitamins during the freezing process.

Of course, the great majority of our foods are processed and 'refined'. 'Refined food' is the ultimate oxymoron. Normally refined means 'better than'. In this context judge for yourself. Next time you have your refined pasta 'healthy lunch' ladies, remember this:

Refined wheat has lost

– at least 75 per cent of its B vitamins
– at least 90 per cent of its mineral content
– at least 98 per cent of its vitamin E
– at least 99 per cent of its fibre.

The refining process has added about 10 per cent to the calorific levels, though.

Other problems associated with our foods in general are:

- Irradiation: it aims to kill the bugs but almost certainly alters the electronic structure of the atoms in the molecules. You are eating a form of genetically modified food, complete with weakened vitamins and minerals.
- Polishes: most fruit is treated with polishes to make it look good. Unfortunately this traps the pesticide residues on the skin underneath. You cannot wash it, yet it was subjected to a dozen chemical sprays. The only answer is to cut off the skin from an apple or pear; but don't you remember being told that was the healthiest part when you were a child?
- Hidden ingredients: sugar, salt, sweeteners, flavours, fillers (e.g. milk fillers), disinfectants. Tasty!
- Fruits have become sweeter. A study of apples showed sugar content had risen by nearly 50 per cent as farmers selected variants to appease supposed sweeter taste demands from the public.

So there you have it. Quite clearly you are better off, as our authorities try to tell you, eating the 'fresh fruit and vegetables' and not wasting money on supplements!

If only you could be sure you were eating quality living food, fresh locally grown fruit and vegetables, organically grown and in season, then you might get some vitamins and minerals from it. Why do some health authorities, professors and doctors take such a misleading and simplistic view? Why is the EU trying to damage my health?

And just consider a few of these points next time someone tells you supplements are useless:

- Virtually every newly diagnosed person who rings our offices is both **nutritionally deficient** and **nutritionally toxic** (see Chapter 6).
- The World Health Authority is quite clear that 50–70 per cent of cancers are caused by poor diet.
- Almost everyone has an acid body due to stress, alcohol, toxins, our lifestyles and the meats we consume. Although we can correct it with the foods we eat, the ones that leave alkaline ash are much 'weaker' than the foods and lifestyle factors that make you acid, so you need vast quantities of them. Minerals control your acidity/alkalinity balance and alkalinity can be achieved far more easily by taking mineral supplements, especially those containing good levels of organic magnesium and potassium. Furthermore many trace minerals like boron, are just not plentiful in our food anymore, yet essential for our well-being. Boron supplementation will not be allowed under the EU directives.
- The US conducted a five-year study of 38,000 people in China, finishing in 1993. It showed that those supplied with beta-carotene, vitamin E and selenium had a 13 per cent reduction in cancers, despite their already supposed healthy diets.
- The French completed the Su. Vi. Max study in Autumn 2003. 17,000 people taking a pill containing zinc, selenium, beta-carotene and vitamins E and C in a random, blind test. During the seven year test there were 31 per cent less men's cancers and 37 per cent less cancer deaths. These supplements work fast!!
- Coenzyme Q10 peaks in your body at puberty and declines as you age, to low levels after age 50. Yet it is essential for proper mitochondrial function, and mitochondria 'go wrong' in cancer. Supplementation can restore levels in a 60-year-old back to where they were in a 20-year-old. American research has proven this. Supplementation has been shown to be far superior than consuming CoQ10-rich foods. However, if the FSA believes it is better to eat the foods, perhaps you'd like to tuck into pancreas, brain, kidneys, liver and heart instead of supplementing.

- The widely recommended daily dose for vitamin E is almost 300 mgs or 400 International Units (IU). If you ate vitamin E rich foods all day you'd be lucky to get to 100 IUs. Moreover, almost all the research studies on vitamin E show anti-cancer effects on a variety of cancers at the 200 mg level (or 300 IUs). The supplements will be limited to RDAs of 15 mgs (20 IUs). Why does the EU not believe its own top scientists?
- Vitamin D is obtained from fish (fish oils) and through the action of sunlight on the skin. How do you get your vitamin D in the UK in the winter?
- B-12 deficiency is on the increase. Estimated to be over 40 per cent of the general population and 73 per cent of vegetarians, older people have a special problem as B-12 is virtually only found in meats, which require an acid medium in the stomach to extract the B-12. As we age our acid production in the stomach declines. B-12 deficiency has been linked to breast cancer, it is linked to lower folate absorption through the intestine and seems to be also linked to the presence of acidophilus (good) and helicobacter pylori (bad). Chlorella is an excellent supplementary source of B-12. The liver stores B-12 and it takes time for a deficiency to show up.

The subject of supplements was covered extensively in *Everything You Need to Know to Help You Beat Cancer* and full reviews are available on www.iconmag.co.uk. To avoid repetition the information is presented in the form of a table, showing you where you can eat your vitamins, the benefits of the vitamin and if you need to supplement and how:

Anti-cancer vitamin or mineral	Daily preventative anti-cancer dose	Benefit	Source
Vitamin A	Female 700 micrograms; male 900 micrograms	Many studies show its cancer-fighting abilities. For example, it protects in breast cancer (Iowa study) and causes remission in leukaemia (Sloan-Kettering). It can be formed in the body from its precursor beta-carotene.	Oily fish are the best source. Cod liver oil supplements.
Beta-carotene	6–25 mgs. Water soluble so take small amounts frequently.	Various studies all link beta-carotene with 30–40 per cent reductions in cancer risk rates. (One study with smokers and people exposed to asbestos suggests it worsens their risks of cancer, though.)	Beta-carotene is the orange pigment in carrots, peppers, apricots and pumpkins. Plus cherries, sweet potato, chicory, spinach, tomato juice and kale.

Anti-cancer vitamin or mineral	Daily preventative anti-cancer dose	Benefit	Source
Vitamin C	1 gm. Water soluble so take small amounts frequently.	Vitamin C boosts the immune system, protects cells and cell walls from attack and, in large doses, helps oxygenate cancer cells (since cancer cells can't use oxygen, this kills them). It also neutralises the toxins from parasites.	Vitamin C is always best taken naturally, and anyway it is plentiful, as it often comes 'packaged' with bioflavonoids and enzymes that help its absorption and action. Best sources are: red peppers, broccoli, papaya, berries, cauliflowers, citrus fruits, potatoes and tomatoes.
Vitamin D	RDA is 5–6 micrograms but anti-cancer level could be five times this. A day in the sun will give you 20–50 times the RDA safely!	Deficiency linked to cancers from prostate to colon. We are only just starting to learn its general importance in cancer from breast to ovarian, prostate to colon. It's really a hormone, not a vitamin. Royal Marsden, UK is providing this to all cancer patients.	Best source is fish oil supplements and via the effect of sunshine on the skin. Dairy can provide a little, but excess dairy depresses its levels.

Anti-cancer vitamin or mineral	Daily preventative anti-cancer dose	Benefit	Source
Vitamin E	400 IU	A crucial vitamin in the fight against cancer, it protects and boosts immune cells. It stops fats damaging the immune system and cells by turning them 'rancid'. Low levels are linked to several cancers. The biggest problem is getting enough, as this vitamin has been the hardest hit by soil depletion.	Give up snack foods and put out a bowl of pumpkin, sunflower and sesame seeds to nibble through the day. Soya, wheatgerm, most nuts (e.g. almonds), whole wheat, whole grains, spinach and eggs are good sources.
Selenium	100–200 (max) micrograms	One of the most important anti-cancer minerals, research has shown its effectiveness in a number of studies. The UK diet is the poorest in Europe for selenium and it is easily destroyed by smoking, fats and oils. One positive effect is that it replaces mercury, lead and some oestrogen-mimics in the body, but then they in turn can replace selenium! Selenium helps the action of vitamin E.	It is found in garlic, tuna and several fish, lobster, onions, broccoli, tomatoes, sunflower seeds, wheatgerm, bran, eggs, brazil nuts and chicken breast.

Anti-cancer vitamin or mineral	**Daily preventative anti-cancer dose**	**Benefit**	**Source**
Lycopene	10–15 mgs	A general immune system booster, but particularly crucial to prostate cancer. One action is to bind to and neutralise fats in the bloodstream.	It is found in tomatoes, tomatoes and especially cooked tomatoes! Harvard Medical School has shown that 7–10 helpings of tomatoes per week (especially cooked), reduce prostate risk by 40 per cent, and symptoms by the same amount. Displaces toxic metals from tissues.

Anti-cancer vitamin or mineral	**Daily preventative anti-cancer dose**	**Benefit**	**Source**
Coenzyme Q10 (ubiquinone)	25–50 mgs	A powerful antioxidant that gets the power stations in your cells running smoothly. These power stations (called mitochondria) work abnormally in cancer cells. CoQ10 also seems to prevent brain cell deterioration (along with omega 3), is important for correct heart function, and helps vitamin E protect the body from free radical attack. CoQ10 declines in production as you age. Long-term supplementation has been proven effective; it can even restore missing energy.	CoQ10 is found in every plant and animal, particularly pancreas, heart, kidney, sardines, salmon, mackerel, beef, spinach, peanuts, soya. However it is best taken as a supplement. Takes three months to build up in body but 50 mgs daily has returned 60-year-olds to levels for twenty-somethings! (Can negatively react with medications for heart and diabetes problems.)
Glutathione	Little need for supplements	A very powerful antioxidant that is produced in all cells of the body. Older people with the highest levels in their bloodstream overcome disease and illness quickest. It works to neutralise fats and free radicals.	Top providers are avocado, asparagus, watermelon, grapefruit, strawberries, raw tomatoes, oranges and boiled potatoes, sprouts, cabbage, cauliflower and broccoli.

Anti-cancer vitamin or mineral	Daily preventative anti-cancer dose	Benefit	Source
B-12	Take chlorella (or B complex)	Essential, and involved in almost every cell and over 300 chemical actions. Deficiency linked to cancers and low folate levels.	Liver, kidney, lean meat, oysters, fish, seafood. Chlorella excellent.
Folic Acid (Vitamin B9)	Take B complex, or 400 micrograms of folate supplement	Essential for the accurate division and replication of DNA. It helps in the development of key enzymes and in the brain function.	Leafy vegetables, avocado, pulses, carrots, melon, apricots, whole wheat. Destroyed by oestrogen, and oestrogen mimics.
Biotin	B complex or 0.3 mgs biotin supplement	Helps the action of immune boosters like vitamin C and helps other B vitamins work. Works with A, B2, B6 and niacin.	Nuts, fruits, whole rice. (N.B. Eggs inhibit absorption; oestrogen destroys it.)
Vitamin K	No maximum level set	Recent research shows an effect in leukaemias and liver cancers at up to 20 times RDA levels. Impossible to eat this much!	Green leafy vegetables, broccoli, supplements.

Anti-cancer vitamin or mineral	Daily preventative anti-cancer dose	Benefit	Source
Acidophilus	Take probiotic supplement	Keeps yeasts and microbes in check; may have anti-cancer action against Helicobacter pylori which is linked to colon cancers, boosts immune system and helps produce biotin.	Simplest to take a supplement to ensure regular presence in intestines. Destroyed by antibiotics, steroids, chemotherapy, acid conditions and chlorinated water.
Omega 3	Take 500 mgs of pure cod liver oil	Numerous anti-cancer studies show it is highly effective. Turns off enzymes that create negative environments in the body. Excellent for brain and general health too.	Long-chain is far more effective than short-chain omega 3. Long-chain is from oily fish and fish oils, short-chain from linseed and flaxseed.

Supplements – the final word

There is a note or two of caution about supplements.

- Multivitamin and mineral pills and tablets are often collections of vitamins and minerals 'stuck' together. If they do not dissolve within 30 minutes in the stomach, they are less likely to be absorbed. It is far better to take a liquid multivitamin and mineral supplement, for example Neways Maximol Classic.
- Following the new EU directives most vitamins sold in the high street will be synthetic, largely coming from the by-products of the petro-chemical industry. There is some evidence that such products are nowhere near as beneficial as the equivalent vitamins from foods.

- Natural vitamins only have to contain 10 per cent from natural sources and these often are not what you would like. B-12 can come from cows' livers, vitamin E (*d*-version) from plants, some natural B vitamins from yeast.
- Minerals are often produced from ground-up rock! The mineral composition is then refined down to leave the desired zinc or selenium but, depending upon the quality of the vitamin/mineral supplement, can have up to 8 per cent of each of a number of unwanted minerals like copper or even arsenic!

Choose your supplement supplier wisely, looking for purity, low levels of toxins and truly natural sources, like pine bark extract or grape seed extract.

PART V

LIVING HEALTH

INTRODUCTION

"Retirement at sixty five is ridiculous. When I was sixty five, I still had pimples".

(George Burns, who laughed into his 100th year!)

Now we arrive at the branches, the foods that actively protect. We have seen the logic of Gerson and Plaskett, the types of food they believe make a difference.

Science shows us that there are particular foods and ingredients that can have a startling effect on your health and this section looks at the important ones. Foods you can add into your diet to make a difference.

Remember though, this is a book on diet. In Everything You Need to Know to Help You Beat Cancer *we covered other important health factors like your attitude to life, your ability to laugh.*

Whatever you do, it is never too late to start building yourself a healthy diet. Start adding these foods into your diet at once.

CHAPTER 18
FOODS THAT ACTIVELY PROTECT

You've cut out the bad guys, boosted your immune system and cleaned up your liver. What else might make a difference?

(i) Fish and fish oils

Nucleic acids

Although the body is quite capable of making nucleic acids at any age, studies have shown that the body can do with a little help. Dr Benjamin Frank (*Nucleic Acid Therapy in Ageing and Degenerative Disease*) showed, nearly thirty years ago, that we need to produce about one to one and a half grams daily of nucleic acid. Dr Frank believed that supplementation was possibly helpful, but that nucleic acid rich foods could retard or even reverse the ageing process.

Top of his list was fish, which he believed should be eaten at least seven times per week. He also suggested freshly made fruit or vegetable juice and good water intake. Apparently **all** his patients benefited from his diet.

Nucleic acid rich foods include fish (especially sardines, anchovies, the Mediterranean staples, and salmon), onions, liver, oatmeal, wheatgerm, spinach, asparagus and mushrooms.

Fresh fish is essential to your diet. Sorry, but no vegetarian will ever convince me otherwise! Fish is a crucial part of the diet of the South East Asians, Okinawans, Eskimos and the Mediterranean peoples. Apart from providing the nucleic acids, fish provides fish oils, which can neutralise free-radicals in the body. Finally and most importantly fish oils contain a number of vitamins and minerals associated with reducing the risk of cancer and crucially contain long-chain omega 3, a vital ingredient in the health of cells, as we showed in Chapter 8.

Fresh, oily fish should be eaten at least three times a week, and daily fish oil supplementation is no bad thing.

Fish oils have been proven to aid general body health, preventing heart disease and dementia, and also to aid cancer prevention and control.

Fish oils contain **omega 3, vitamin A** and **vitamin D,** and most contain good levels of **selenium** and some **vitamin E**. These five have all been shown to have very active roles in beating cancer.

You may have read a lot about omega 3, omega 6, and essential fatty acids. As if that wasn't enough, omega 3 can be found in short-chain and long-chain forms. So it is worth saying right up front that **omega 3 long-chain oils are the good guys**; in fact, it is doubtful that your body can gain full benefit from the short chain version, alpha linolenic acid, which is normally obtained from seeds. Some conversion occurs between short-chain and long-chain but it is restricted.

Long-chain omega 3 oils only come from oil-rich fish. Table A shows the relative benefits of various cold, salt-water fish.

The origins of these long-chain polyunsaturated fats are the microscopic algae and plankton that the fish feed on. Sadly, of course, fish farming methods may mean less consumption of these vital nutrients. This is why the best fish is **'deep-sea caught'.**

TABLE A	Lipid content	Omega 3
Oil		
Cod Liver	100.0	20.0
Fish		
Mackerel	16.1	2.0
Herring	13.2	2.0
Salmon	11.0	2.3
Sprat	9.9	2.4
Rock Salmon (dogfish)	9.7	2.3
Sardines	9.2	2.5
Crab	5.5	1.2
Tuna	4.6	1.6

Volumes in gms per 100gms of edible portion

Short-chain omega 3 oils are found in flaxseed, rapeseed and linseed amongst others.

To understand the importance of omega 3 in our bodily functions it is necessary to understand the development of man. In the era of dinosaurs, early forms of homosapiens would emerge from their caves and often the main source of nourishment was the brain left behind in the carcass of a dinosaur's victim. The brain, indeed your brain, contains high levels of omega 3. Our diets were originally 2:1, omega 3:omega 6. By the 1900s that had become 1:1. Now the average New York female has a 1:25 or even 1:50 diet. Supplementing with evening primrose oil for menstrual problems worsens this. Omega 6 (linoleic acid) is found in sunflower, sesame and safflower oils; in its gamma form it is found in evening primrose oil and borage – but it is extremely doubtful that anyone need supplement with omega 6, given modern diets!

Omega 3 is thought to be linked to our intelligence; children who take regular supplementation were shown in US studies to have IQs 11 per cent higher than those that didn't. A deficiency of omega 3 has also been clearly linked to Alzheimer's. A great number of recent studies have argued for its crucial role in cancer prevention and cure, from colon, to prostate, to breast and oesophageal cancers.

Whilst omega 3, omega 6 and indeed most fats find their way into a general **'oil pool'** of fatty acids inside the body, only long-chain omega 3 can turn this into a positive benefit.

Indeed excessive levels of omega 6 in the body's 'oil pool' have been deemed harmful, signalling heart attacks, headaches and asthma amongst other illnesses. The percentage of omega 6 in the 'oil pool' is 30 per cent in Greenland, 50 per cent in Japan, 60 per cent in the Mediterranean and 80 per cent in the USA (*The Lancet* 1999). Clearly it is safer to keep it to 50 per cent or lower.

In Chapter 8 we saw how omega 3 could turn off an enzyme (called Cox-2) which hormonally produces 'bad' eicosanoids.

There are two strong implications for eicosanoids:

Firstly, that eicosanoids provide the last link in the chain, which communicates messages from your brain to localised cells. Put simply, if your brain feels stressed, this will be communicated (via cortisol from the adrenals, for example) to the nuclear envelope in your breast cells and so your breast cells will be 'stressed' and, with this, increase the risks of cancer.

Secondly, eicosanoids and Cox-2, play a role directly in the cellular pathways involved in malignancy.

It is known that eicosanoids play a key role in cell signalling, primarily in oxidative pathways. Cox-2 plays a role in cell growth, and human tumour cells have high levels of Cox-2. Cox-2 also plays a key role in the synthesis of prostaglandins, which are found mainly in inflammatory and immune cells. Whilst prostaglandins and some other eicosanoids bring about tissue responses such as wound repair and inflammation, in excess they are implicated totally in many modern diseases e.g. atherosclerosis, rheumatic diseases, Alzheimer's and cancers.

Cox-2 levels are high in 85 per cent of colon cancers (Dubois, Vanderbilt), and also in breast cancer. Work is underway on drugs, which block Cox-2. **But why take drugs when the fundamental answer lies in increasing your intake of fish oils?** The *International Journal of Cancer* (March 2002) reports on 250 women with breast cancer and the findings that **women who are cancer free have much higher omega 3 fatty acid levels in their breast tissue!**

There are some points to watch for. Much coastal fish contains toxins, especially mercury. Many fish oils contain high levels of toxic dioxins, so check with the manufacturer and only buy fish oils with low dioxin levels. Best of all is deep-sea caught natural oily fish. But it is wise to ensure you have good selenium levels in your diet to displace any mercury that might be present, although fish does have built-in selenium too!

The issue of mercury is much referred to. In France, mercury must be transported in double thickness container lorries with a police escort, and we put it in our teeth! Worse, it is in over 70 common vaccines, and both contain far more mercury than fish.

Cancer-fighting vitamins and minerals

Vitamin A is a fat-soluble vitamin, part of a family of compounds including retinol. It helps boost the immune system and there are a number of impressive research studies supporting its effectiveness in the fight against cancer.

Vitamin A cannot be synthesised in the body and must be taken in with food as retinol or in its precursor form, beta-carotene.

Fish and fish oils except for cod liver oil contain significant quantities of both vitamin A and vitamin D. Cod liver oil, unless supplemented, contains no vitamin D.

TABLE B	Vitamin A (mcgs)	Vitamin D (mcgs)
Cod liver oil	2	–
Mackerel	45	5
Herring	44	19
Salmon	13	8
Sprat	60	13
Rock Salmon (dogfish)	9.4	–
Sardines	–	11
Tuna	26	7.2

per 100 gms edible portion

The first link between human cancer and vitamin A was in 1941 (Abelsetal), with low plasma vitamin A levels linked to gastro-intestinal cancers. Later studies (Moon et al), showed prevention of squamous cell skin carcinoma, lowered levels of mesothelioma (de Klerk), oral leukoplakias (Stitch). Indeed there is evidence of a link of vitamin A with cancers of the breast, prostate, stomach, colon/rectum and upper digestive tract. A study in 1993 of 90,000 breast cancer patients in New England, linked vitamin A to decreased tumour activity. Another study at the Memorial Sloan-Kettering Institute linked vitamin A supplementation to an 80 per cent remission in leukaemia.

The anti-cancer effects of retinols are thought to be due to their promotion of cell differentiation, inhibition of cell proliferation and the enhancement of the immune system. But beware of taking too much cod liver oil or vitamin enriched fish oil. As a fat-soluble vitamin, vitamin A can build up in the body and particularly the liver, and over time excess can cause toxicity.

Fish and fish oils also have high levels of **vitamin D.** An RDA for vitamin D has never been accurately defined, although an intake of five micrograms was thought to be sufficient for people under 50 based on studies over 50 years old in preventing rickets. However the last five years have shown that vitamin D plays an important anti-cancer role and levels of five times this are appropriate. The Royal Marsden Cancer Centre in the UK is giving vitamin D supplements to patients, such is the importance they place on this vitamin. The only other major 'source' of which is sunshine on the skin (although dairy contains a little).

Vitamin D has a molecular structure similar to steroids; in fact, cholesterol is a precursor for both and the truth is that it is more like a hormone than a vitamin.

Sunlight acts on the skin causing the photo-conversion of a form of cholesterol into vitamin D3. However, in our polluted cities, humans with their indoor jobs and multiple layers of clothing can be D3 deficient.

Black people have a higher incidence of cancers like prostate and colon cancer. It is thought that their skin pigmentation prevents vitamin D being made, causing them a deficiency of this important cancer protector.

Ingestion of vitamin D is therefore necessary in these cases and crucial in some cases of cancer.

D3 is metabolised by the liver to make 'circulating D' which in turn is broken down by the kidneys to two D 'active ingredients' which then bind at receptor sites on target organs to make things happen.

In May 2002, The Howard Hughes Medical Institute heard how vitamin D protects against colon cancer by helping to detoxify a highly carcinogenic bile acid (lithocholic acid) produced in response to high fat diets.

It has become increasingly clear since 1980 that D3 plays a role linked to mineral metabolism, particularly in the blood system and in cell differentiation and proliferation, including reactions with keratinocytes, cancer cells and in insulin secretion. Thus it is linked to eicosanoid signalling, as was covered in Part I. (Bouillon, Okamura and Norman, *Endocrinology Review* 16 1995; Norman, University of California 2000).

D3 is found in cow's milk in small quantities but the high calcium and protein content may inhibit its action. D3 is one of the most important biological regulators of calcium metabolism, stimulating its absorption from food and monitoring calcium and phosphate levels causing calcium to be stored in the bones, thus preventing osteoporosis. Too much vitamin D can produce hypercalcaemia although a fortnight's holiday in the sun can produce 10,000–20,000 IUs per day without any harm to the individual.

Selenium is a vital mineral in your protection against cancer. It is an antioxidant that works in conjunction with vitamin E, which is also found in fish and fish oils in small amounts. In a recent study, selenium appeared to reduce mortality from all cancers, and particularly the incidence of lung, colorectal and prostate (Merck). Poor selenium levels have been linked to cancers of the stomach and breast.

TABLE C	**Selenium (mcgs)**
Lobster	130
Tuna	57
Rock Salmon (dogfish)	55
Mussels	51
Plaice	37
Herring	35
Cod	28
Salmon	24

It appears to work with vitamin E in membrane protection especially of immune cells, and works via gluthatione peroxidase, an enzyme that neutralises hydroperoxides formed from fats.

The population of the UK has the lowest selenium intake in Europe (possibly since we consume far less garlic and fish both of which can contain good levels of selenium).

Fish and fish oils also have small levels of **vitamin E**, a vitamin that is increasingly depleted in our vegetables and which plays a significant anti-cancer role.

Finally, fish is an excellent source of nucleic acids and as we mentioned in Chapter 7, these have been proven helpful in anti-ageing processes.

N.B. *There has been some recent research in the *American Journal of Clinical Medicine* (Nov. 2002) that fish oils may be dangerous to certain diabetics. At all times we suggest you take proper medical advice.

It is hard to understand, for example, how the usual Health Authority advice of eating five helpings of fruit and vegetables, or a balanced diet could possibly replicate the omega 3 levels our ancestors had in their bodies, or even give us levels of long-chain omega 3 necessary to ensure full health. A good level of fresh fish consumption and then some supplementation would seem essential for all of us. However we are failing to do either in the UK.

For example, between 1900 and 1950 cod liver oil production was regularly 75,000 tonnes per annum. Now it is just 20,000 tonnes.

(ii) Garlic

Garlic crops up time and time again in the fight against cancer, whether we are looking at Asian diets, or Mediterranean diets, glycoproteins or yeast control.

Garlic has strong anti-cancer benefits. For example, it seems to restrict the blood supply to cancer tumours and thus stops them growing.

Garlic is particularly protective in stomach, gastric and colon cancers, and across several epidemiological studies, it has been linked to reduced rates of a wider range of cancers, from lung to oesophageal. For example, in the Iowa Women's Health Study (USA Steinmetz 1994) of 127 foods, tested with 41,387 women, garlic was the only fruit or vegetable that produced an effect; one or more servings of fresh garlic a week was linked with 35 per cent less colon cancer and 50 per cent less distal colon cancer.

In a 1998 study in China (You et al) people taking large quantities of garlic every day (up to 60 gms per day!) had less than half the cancers of those taking only a little.

The bad news is that **fresh, chopped or squeezed garlic is essential.** Cooking ruins the effect and, in tests, some garlic pills are pretty useless.

Although many reports talk about the active ingredient being allicin, other anti-cancer agents appear to be produced on cutting or crushing. Other ingredients include alliin and the enzyme allinase. It is possible that allicin works as an antioxidant, and it is certainly effective in reducing blood cholesterol levels. Allicin is also a very strong natural weapon against microbial infection, particularly bacteria, viruses, yeasts and intestinal amoeba. By eradicating them it could help the fight against cancer in several indirect ways, as we saw in Chapter 16 – allicin interferes with enzymes necessary for the growth of these infectious organisms and also enhances a liver enzyme, which detoxifies aflatoxins before they cause damage.

Allicin thus wards off infection and allows the body's natural defences to be stronger. Allinase seems to promote this action and in tests, allicin has been shown to inhibit cancers of the breast, liver and colon. Allicin appears to bind to breast cell receptor sites preventing the action of cancer agents. Prostate cells exposed to the garlic chemical SAMC grow at only 25 per cent of the normal rate.

Garlic also seems to protect the body against the side effects of radiotherapy, particularly DNA and chromosome damage.

Professor Wargovich of the University of Texas has been working with two other active ingredients: dialylsuphide and S-allylcysteine. These have been shown to reduce animal cancers by 50 to 75 per cent and, in another test on animal cells, to totally protect against a deliberate attempt to induce a particularly virulent oesophageal cancer.

Finally, there are three other possible routes for cancer protection:

- Some garlic contains quite good levels of selenium. Indeed, hybrids of garlic are being produced which are selenium rich and these have been shown to be especially effective against breast cancer.
- Garlic, as we will see in the next section, contains glycoproteins which help cancer fighters get into cells and toxins get out.
- Garlic also contains good levels of tryptophan, which is the precursor of serotonin, which in turn is the precursor of melatonin. Melatonin, as we saw earlier, is an excellent and very powerful neutraliser of free radicals. Precursors are known to stimulate its production, even in people of advancing years.

You will all be pleased to know that the EU is not about to ban garlic. If they did, I'm sure the French would create a real stink!

(iii) Glycoproteins and polysaccharides

Nobel Prizes

Four Nobel Prizes for Medicine in recent years (1994, 1999, 2000 and 2001) have been won with research on how cells communicate, and importance to our health and well-being.

Whilst one of them was specifically concerned with the brain and how nerve cells communicate through chemicals with each other (Arvid Carlsson et al 2000), the other three were concerned with communications to cells around the body and all had implications for cancer prevention and treatment.

In 1994 Gilman and Rodbell won for their discovery of 'G-proteins and the role of these in signal transduction in cells'. Basically they investigated how localised cells handle signal substances from glands, nerves and other tissues to make changes.

In 1999 Gunter Blöbel and his team looked at how proteins have specific protein signals built into them so that they reach the correct destinations.

And by 2001 Hartwell, Hunt and Nurse had won for showing an understanding on the cellular messages involved in the cell cycle – its growth and division into two identical daughter cells – and how mistakes might result in a cancer development.

These protein messages often involve carbohydrate molecules, or sugars, and so it is common in the USA to call them 'super-carbs' or monosaccharides (which is actually wrong as most are polysaccharides). In fact most are a combination of 'sugars' and peptides (small proteins of less than 30 amino acids in length). I prefer the generic term 'glycoproteins', the word first coined for this hot topic. Several aspects of glycoproteins are important.

Blöbel sought to understand a genetic mystery. When your DNA string is read and the code says you should have blue eyes or blond hair, how does the message get to the right place?

As a foetus in the womb, each of us started out with a fused cell from our parents that multiplied at an incredibly rapid rate. As we covered earlier, around day 56 something (largely thought to be a message from the pancreas) tells these cells, called stem cells, to turn into eye cells or hair cells, and to stop dividing so rapidly and instead to adopt a normal cell cycle.

The interest for cancer scientists is that cancer cells resemble stem cells but do not seem to have received the signal to differentiate.

Blöbel found that the messages sent out contained little 'post-codes' directing the message to the hair cells or the eye cells.

Furthermore he discovered that these signals contain the ability to go through the cell membrane and so influence the mechanism of the cell inside.

Cell membranes – barriers to health?

Cell membranes are largely made up of fats or lipids and protein. If you think of each molecule as a pin, with a pinhead, alternately pointing in opposite directions but in a neat line, you will have a picture of a healthy membrane. Messages can thus slip in between the pins. It is the role of glycoproteins to encourage this 'neatness' and thus allow the messages through. Healthy cells allow toxins out, and certain cancer 'protectors' in.

The problem comes when the pins are not in this neat format and are fused or damaged, not allowing anything through. Worse, sometimes modest amounts of carbohydrate are bonded to the membranes blocking their transmitting power further.

Where tumour cells have this carbohydrate, it is used to bind to other cells and cause them to turn rogue too, hence causing metastasis. Killer cells in your immune system look out for these carbohydrate-bonded sites, but if the membranes are imperfect they can hide and the killer cells may not be able to attack the rogue cell or, worse, even recognise it.

Blöbel's work focused on what happens when there are errors in the signals, while Hartwell et al focused on what happens when the cell cycle goes haywire.

What this means to you and me

The need for healthy signalling and message flow has led to a focus on glycoproteins.

Professor Gilbon-Garber has shown, for example, that the invasive process of bacteria, viruses and indeed cancer cells which involves the above 'bonding' process to membranes, can be inhibited by glycoproteins in mother's milk.

Because these molecules (from mother's milk, saliva and semen) used in her experiments are all-natural, no side effects occurred.

And furthermore, natural breast milk contains important agents affording protection against infection. Scientists have clearly shown that children who are breastfed are ill less than those fed on substitute products. So it could be that glycoprotein 'drugs' could clear up the membranes and have wider protective effects.

In a recent Danish research study, breastfeeding doesn't just make babies healthier, it was found to make them cleverer too.

In a study of 9,000 Danish women and men, those who were breastfed to month nine scored significantly higher in IQ tests later in life, than those not breastfed past month two.

Scientists believe breast milk contains nutrients like glycoproteins that nourish brain cells and protect against infection.

This has important implications. 'Drugs' could be based on natural substances, with no side effects. But why make drugs? Polysaccharides are all around us.

So where can I get them? And fast!

A number of naturally occurring substances have already been identified as having high polysaccharide content.

Not surprisingly one was **medicinal mushrooms**. Reishi, maiitake, cordyceps and oyster mushrooms all contain beta-glucan polysaccharide. Cancer Research UK reported recently that Japanese mushroom pickers have 40 per cent of the cancer rates of the rest of the population. (They obviously scrump!).

Other natural sources of these essential glycoproteins are:

Aloe vera, Noni juice;
Arabinogalactins – found in carrots, leeks, radishes, pears, red wine, coconut meat, tomatoes, curcumin and echinacea, corn;
Brans – slow cooked oatmeal, whole barley, brown rice;
Breast milk;
Garlic;
Pectins – apples, pears and citrus fruit eaten whole;
Psyllium.

The interesting factor is the universality of the discovery. All cells seem to positively respond to glycoproteins, whether they are human, yeast, plants or animals.

Even tiny amounts of these sugars – or lack of them – have a profound effect. One polysaccharide 'mix', Ambrotose, is used by a number of cancer clinics to enhance the immune system.

One integrated cancer expert we spoke to said that glycoproteins would be more important than all discoveries like vitamin C, B-17 and genistein added together!

You most definitely should ensure you incorporate the above foods into your diet. Despite all the Nobel Prizes, any natural supplements for glycoproteins are unlikely to be on the new EU approved lists as the directive currently stands!

(iv) B-17

B-17 or amygdalin is a naturally occurring vitamin. In fact it is slightly wrong to think of it as a single product like, say, vitamin C. There is a group of approximately 14 products which are water-soluble, and found naturally in over 1,200 species of plant in the world. Every area of the world supporting vegetation has such plants.

The products are often described as nitrilosides or beta-cyanogenetic glucosides and there are at least 800 foods common in worldwide diets that are nitrilosidic. Sadly in the UK we are eating less and less of those that were indigenous to our shores.

These foods include:

Alfalfa sprouts, bamboo shoots, mung bean sprouts;
Barley, buckwheat, maize, millet;
Blackberries, currants, cassava, cranberries, gooseberries, loganberries, quince, raspberries, strawberries, yams;
Brown rice, fava beans, lentils and many pulses like kidney beans, lima beans and field beans;
Flaxseed, linseed;
Pecan nuts, macadamia nuts, cashews, walnuts;
Watercress, sweet potato;
Almonds and the **seeds** of lemons, limes, cherries, apples, apricots, prunes, plums and pears.

The consumption of barley, buckwheat and millet has given way to refined wheats whilst, as we discussed before, our consumption of pulses like lentils has declined markedly. Watercress consumption is in decline in the UK, as is our consumption of our own pears, cherries, plums and apples. We no longer have the volumes of raspberries, gooseberries, blackcurrants and nut trees, and certainly not the hedgerows of blackberries, or quince that we had in the middle-ages. We are truly neglecting the foods that kept us healthy.

Primitive tribes around the world still base their diets around B-17 rich foods. Cassava, papaya, yam, sweet potato in the tropics; unrefined rice in the Far East; seeds and nuts in the Himalayas; the salmon-berry eaten by Eskimos, or the arrow-grass of the arctic tundra feeding the caribou.

Nutritionist and scientists alike studied the various tribes. Sir Robert McCarrison in the 1920s and Dr John Dark twenty years later failed to find a single case of cancer amongst the Hunzas, the tribes of West Pakistan. V. Stefansson found the same with the Eskimos and wrote *Cancer: Disease of Civilisation?* as a result. Dr M. Navarro of Santo Thomas, University of Manilla, noticed the same with the Philippine population who ate cassava, wild rice, wild beans, berries and fruits of all kinds. Dr Albert Schweitzer noted the same in Gabon "this absence of cancer seemed to be due to the difference of nutrition in the natives compared to the Europeans". Their diet was centred around sorghum, cassava, millet and maize.

Studies of the consumption of B-17 varied from Dark's finding that the Hunzas consumed at least 150–250mgs per day, to Dean Burk, Head of Cytochemistry Department of the National Cancer Institute in the USA in the seventies writing that the Modoc Indians in North America consumed over 8,000 mgs per day!

We leave these foods aside at our peril.

Cancer treatments

It is worth noting that B-17 has been used as a cancer treatment for a number of years. Amygdalin was first isolated in 1830 and used as an anti-cancer agent in Russia as early as 1845. But it was reborn by the father/son team Ernst Krebs senior and junior, who isolated a purified form of the active ingredient (calling it laetrile) and, with others in the late fifties to seventies, sought to explain its action.

Cancer cells differ in a number of ways from normal cells. One difference as we have said earlier is that the mitochondria, or power stations, do not use oxygen to produce energy, and need a whole different energy system and a different set of chemicals (enzymes). In a cancer cell there is a unique enzyme called glucosidase which breaks down B-17 into hydrogen cyanide (which kills it) and benzaldehyde (an analgesic). In normal cells, where glucosidase is virtually non-existent, another enzyme, rhodinase, renders the B-17 harmless. Critics talk about B-17 containing cyanide, but the truth is that so does vitamin B-12 which is universally present in our bodies and no one complains about that. Meanwhile, the proponents clearly believe B-17 is a seek and destroy missile targeting only the cancer cell mitochondria.

Well, maybe. Every day you produce several hundred cancer cells. Get them early with a rich B-17 diet and this could be true. However, as cancers develop they often form protective protein coats around the cells to ward off the immune system. We referred to these membranes under the heading of glycoproteins. These protein coats will protect the tumours from B-17 too.

Various cancer clinics have thus developed 'therapy packages'; these include bromelain (from pineapple), papain (from papaya) and two pancreatic enzymes trypsin and chymotrypsin to break down this protein coat, plus vitamins A, E and B complex, plus high dose vitamin C and high dose minerals.

The difficulty then becomes, "which bit worked?" Having personally talked to leading B-17 therapy users in the USA and Europe, none doubts its efficacy, but all felt it was not as potent as high dose vitamin C, and that clearly a significant contribution was being made by the other participants in the therapy package.

Laetrile has shown effectiveness against cancer cells *in vitro*, and in rats and mice. Even the NCI, which is negative about laetrile, reports that by the late seventies over 70,000 cancer patients had been treated with laetrile and there are copious case histories on its effectiveness. Dr Contreras of the Oasis of Hope Hospital in Mexico is one of the foremost advocates of B-17 therapy. He has dubbed it 'nature's chemotherapy', and uses it on all cancer treatments but notes that it does not work for brain tumours, sarcomas or liver cancer.

Krebs recommended eating ten apricot seeds per day for life as a preventative measure (the seeds, or kernels, have the highest levels of B-17); cancer treatments use four to six 500 mg tablets per day or intravenous injections.

One issue is overdosing. **A maximum of five kernels at any one time in a two-hour period is recommended for preventers,** and cancer treatments have to be properly supervised. I met a gentleman in Australia who had prostate cancer and had been to a speech on B-17. He was taking 35 kernels for breakfast and wondered why he felt sluggish and livery!! Excess B-17 and cyanide by-products have been known to build up in the liver. Each of us has different liver detoxing capacities and the cancer patient has an already impaired liver. Cyanide poisoning of the liver can result if excess is consumed by someone with an impaired liver. **1gm of vitamin B-17 is the maximum recommended dose to be taken at any one time and the US Nutrition Almanac recommends a maximum of 35 seeds per day.**

Foods containing B-17 are to be recommended in any preventative diet, and anybody reviewing the list will see that it has foods in common with several of the other preventative lists in this book and they contain a wonderful array of vitamins, minerals, oils and fibre to protect us all.

Having read the original research on B-17 treatments we find the 'evidence' against laetrile almost non-existent, whilst there are clearly worthy claims for its effectiveness. We simply do not understand the logic of a government Health Authority, the FDA, concluding that it simply doesn't work and so moving to ban the interstate shipments of apricot kernels and planting of bitter almond trees! Even my mother's Asda 'iced log' (a cake) in the UK, contained 11 per cent apricot kernel paste! Presumably this cannot be moved between California and Nevada!

To the major UK Charity who claims on its website that, "*if laetrile worked, surely it would have been developed by a pharmaceutical company by now*", we say this is an appallingly poor piece of patient support. And to be as cynical as the charity in question, why would a pharmaceutical company invest millions in B-17 when it cannot be patented and, if shown to be effective, would remove the market for its other products?!

(v) Acid and alkali foods

Acid producers

Your body's cells need a slightly alkaline environment to work at maximum efficiency, as does your immune system. A pH, for those of you who did O Level science, of 7.2 to 7.4 is the aim. But certain foods after ingestion make your body very acid, as do many lifestyle factors like smoking and stress.

Protein is extremely acid-forming because it contains sulphur compounds, as do wheat, rye and many processed foods. The end product after digestion is sulphuric acid.

Excess sodium makes the inside of our cells very acid too, as we saw in Chapter 3. And anything that inhibits magnesium, blocks the cell pump and makes cells more acid.

The worst offenders are (in decreasing 'offence' order):

> Liver, crab, shellfish, scallops, all meats, fried foods, most fish, eggs, crisps, salted peanuts, snack food, processed meat, smoked fish, sauces, vinegars, mustard, chocolate, salt, spirits, refined wheat and other refined food like pasta, rice, noodles, fizzy soft drinks, oranges, tomatoes, tea, dairy and wine.

Stress, lack of sleep, smoke, alcohol and other lifestyle factors also make the body acid, so the process of trying to alkalise the body is an uphill battle.

The biochemical action of the 'alkalisers' is largely provided by their minerals, not their vitamins, and by the body's digestion system which produces an alkaline ash in response to their consumption.

The best alkalisers, by and large, are fruit and vegetables. Once digested and oxidised they provide potassium and hydroxyl ions in the environment surrounding your cells. The potassium is pumped into the cell, and sodium is pumped out in exchange reducing the metabolic acidity. The hydroxyl ions which are negative, pull positive hydrogen ions out of the cell to form water further reducing the acidity inside the cells. Apples, apple juice and apple cider vinegar are a good place to start when planning to alkalise your cells.

You can eat to beat cancer by focussing more on the following, which are the best alkaline producers:

> Apples, cooked spinach, fresh ginger, freshly prepared juices, garlic, kale, dates, figs and raisins, soya, soya beans, whole brown rice, papaya, watercress, lemons, beetroot, parsnips, grapes, carrots, celery, all berries and cherries, asparagus and cranberries.

Beware: Citrus fruit juices can generate extremely aggressive cleansing elimination and cause aggravation of symptoms.

(vi) Nuts and other good oils

In Chapter 5 we looked at how bad fats and oils were for you, except for monounsaturated oils.

Basically there are only really two sorts of fats/oils – saturated and unsaturated. The unsaturated ones can be mono or poly 'unsaturated'. In the Far East polyunsaturated oils like soya oil and sunflower oil are used. However, these are pure (unrefined, unhydrogenated) and so have kept all their nourishment unlike many polyunsaturated oils in the West; they are almost solely used for cooking and then only in trace amounts; and the cooking method of extremely intensive but rapid heating does not produce dangerous free radicals. By contrast in the West we refine, hydrogenate and generally ruin our sunflower oils, and our frying methods just encourage the production of free radicals in our bodies.

The best oils as we mentioned earlier are monounsaturated oils.

Most remarkably, monounsaturated oils have the ability to actually neutralise the free radicals produced by saturated fats, and this is one reason why diets high in olive oil, for example, are thought to be 'protective' and healthier. Again this really is an example of how you can eat to beat cancer.

Monounsaturated oils tend to lower harmful low-density lipoprotein (LDL) and cholesterol levels and the best, for example cold pressed olive oil, provides a range of protective phyto-chemicals and phenols.

Monounsaturated oils are also a good source of vitamin E.
Sources of monounsaturated fat:

Olive oil	73%
Rapeseed oil	60%
Hazelnuts	50%
Almonds	35%
Cashews	28%
Brazils	26%
Sesame seeds	20%
Pumpkin seeds	16%

Mediterranean diets are high in olive oil, nut oils and seeds. And this is one reason the population can cope with higher levels of animal fats. (Another reason is tomatoes – just like monounsaturated fats, lycopene can actually bind to and neutralise free radicals and fats in the bloodstream.)

(vii) Isoflavones

Isoflavones or phytoestrogens are widely found all over the world in herbs, plants and vegetables. Phytoestrogens are similar but not identical in chemical composition to oestrogen; their action in the human body is much weaker than the hormone.

One source is soya. Many learned people write about soya and become confused between possible problems with soy, or soya, and possible problems with isoflavones. So let's see if we can clear this up.

Isoflavones and phytoestrogens are very protective to humans and have been thus in both the East and West for thousands of years.

Isoflavones and phytoestrogens have been consumed in the West in broad beans, peas, flageolet and lentils; or chickpeas and hummus; or in red clover (the herb of Hippocrates) and similar herbs; and from fruits (citrus isoflavones).

Cancer Research UK contributed to a study which looked at soya consumption and cancer in Eastern women. Women who consumed the highest amounts had 60 per cent fewer cancers than those who ate the least.

Genistein, one of the active ingredients of soya is also a phytoestrogen, and so it mimics human oestrogen, but unlike the latter it doesn't encourage cancer to spread. All cells have receptor sites on them; human oestrogen can work with cancer to act on healthy receptor sites turning the next cell rogue too. Genistein and other isoflavones, for example red clover isoflavones or citrus isoflavones, stop this by blocking the adjacent healthy receptor site.

Ingredients in soya, like garlic, have also been shown to cut off the blood supply to tumours. Fermented soya products have a less effective action. You should also beware of mass-market soy sauces as they have high sugar and salt content. Shoyu and Tamari, brewed in oak casks are more natural but still high in salt, albeit sea salt.

It is possible that the soya plant, per se, may have some negatives. Let us look at the usual claims. Soya is definitely an incomplete protein and lacks vitamin B-12.

It does contain high levels of protein and oils and these can create problems for cancer sufferers on more extreme therapies, where even modest levels of fat and protein are forbidden. As we saw earlier this was Dr Max Gerson's reason for rejecting it.

Charlotte Gerson says it has high levels of aluminium (it is roughly the same as in milk), much of it is GM tainted (true), and high levels of phytic acid which would limit mineral uptake. Again she does not want this as her patients, often extreme cases, are on a high mineral therapy. All green beans and pulses are thus excluded from the therapy. Plaskett feels this argument is too simplistic, and he allows soya for hormonally responsive cancers, like breast cancers, where the protective phytoestrogens are helpful.

Soya itself does cause allergic reactions in the West, but that is to be expected. It is a 'rich' food and we have only been consuming it for 40 years, so soya should only be consumed in moderation and if any allergic reactions occur it should be stopped immediately.

Red clover, the herb of Hippocrates, has a long history of use as a medicinal herb. It's an excellent blood purifier that gradually cleanses the bloodstream and corrects deficiencies in the circulatory system. But among classic herbalists, it is probably best known as a herb for treating cancer and is found as a central ingredient in a number of herbal anti-cancer formulas, including the Hoxsey formula, Jason Winter's tea, and Essiac tea.

Many USA doctors, the FDA and even 'new-school' herbalists, have dismissed red clover as useless in dealing with cancer. Now researchers at the National Cancer Institute have confirmed that there are indeed anti-tumour properties in red clover. One, genistein, has the ability to prevent tumours from developing the blood supplies they need to survive, thus starving and killing them.

Genistein is the same biochemical considered to be the main beneficial ingredient in soya. But red clover has a significant advantage over soya, as it contains about ten times the level found in soya of all four main oestrogen isoflavones, including daidzein and genistein.

In addition to isoflavones, red clover contains another class of anti-cancer phytoestrogens, compounds called coumestans, for example, biochanin and formononetin. Consuming red clover isoflavones results in higher blood levels of daidzein and genistein, moderate blood levels of formononetin. Soy consumption does not result in any increase in biochanin or formononetin in the blood.

Asian women, who have far, far less cancers than Western women, have up to a thousand times the isoflavone levels in their bloodstreams when compared to their Western equivalents, and many studies have concluded that this is a vital and protective factor.

The fact is that in the West our protective isoflavones and phytoestrogens levels have fallen dramatically as we turn away from the foods (vegetables, pulses, fruits) and herbs that protected us. Our need is to build our Western phytoestrogens **back** into our diets, not merely resort to some 'trendy' Eastern food to which we might be allergic. Isoflavones and phytoestrogens do protect, that's a fact, be they citrus isoflavones (being used with success for brain tumours), in red clover (effective with several cancers and being studied with breast cancer at the Royal Marsden) or genistein used by Plaskett and a number of clinics in hormonally driven cancer treatments.

(viii) Ellagic acid

Ellagic acid is a proven anti-carcinogen, anti-mutagen and anti-cancer initiator.

Dr Daniel Nixon at the Hollings Cancer Institute, at the Medical University of South Carolina (MUSC) began studying ellagic acid in 1993.

Recent published data from MUSC includes the findings that:

- Ellagic acid slows the growth of abnormal colon cells.
- Ellagic acid has antibacterial and anti-viral properties. It can prevent HPV infected cells developing, and cervical cells infected with HPV experience apoptosis (normal cell death).
- It increases the rate of metabolism of carcinogens and prevents the development of cancer cells.
- It affects and inhibits the action of arylamines, known as potent carcinogens.
- As a powerful antioxidant it neutralises the affects of aflatoxins produced by parasites within the body.

And all this seems to come from eating just **one cup of red raspberries per day!**

Initial studies and clinical tests have shown that ellagic acid can protect the *p53* gene. This gene has the ability to rebuild damaged DNA under normal conditions. But as part of cancer development it becomes ‘switched off’. There is some evidence that this is a factor in breast, prostate, pancreas, skin, cervical and colon cancers. Ellagic acid also seems to form ‘joints’ with DNA by binding to sites which would otherwise be attacked by mutagens or carcinogens.

MUSC are now hoping to conduct a double blind test on humans over a two-year period, studying its effect on cervical cancer in particular.

Preliminary studies are extremely positive with even small concentrations inhibiting growth within 48 hours and causing apoptosis (cell death) within 72 hours.

Ellagic acid, an extremely stable polyphenol, is found in some 46 different fruits and nuts, for example pomegranate, red raspberries, blackberries, strawberries, blueberries, cranberries, pecans and walnuts.

Of course you can now buy supplements – but why not eat the above? You only need half to one cup full according to Dr Nixon.

(ix) Red wine, green tea

As you read this book you will have spotted several mentions of red wine. It has a protective effect on the pancreas, it contains arabinogalactins, a type of glycoprotein, and it contains catechins and resveratrol, both strong antioxidants. White wine does not have the same effect because, by and large, these properties come from the red grape skin and seeds. (Red grape seeds are being tested as an anti-cancer agent.) The fermenting process seems to concentrate these benefits. The French and Italians drink their wine with their meals and the alcohol in the blood actually has a 'dissolving' effect on the fat.

Similarly the Chinese drink green tea, their cup of antioxidants, and their balancer of acids. With it the Thais take lemongrass, which is about 100 times more powerful than betacarotene when fresh.

In Britain we used to drink honey drinks. Antioxidant and anti-microbial (the honey contains ingredients that prevented bacteria attaching on to the natural sugars in the hive). What is the antioxidant drink of the Western world now? Certainly not coffee, or coca cola!

(x) Algae

The earliest life forms; over 30,000 species inhabit the earth where there is a natural water supply. At one extreme are microscopic blue-green algae, at the other 150 foot long strands of kelp.

Probably the best known are spirulina and chlorella, both having many properties in common, although unlike other algae chlorella has a nucleus.

They are excellent sources of vitamins and minerals, enzymes (including digestive enzymes) and amino acids (with all eight essential acids). However, they have notable other benefits.

Spirulina and chlorella are both excellent sources of polysaccharides (see section on Glycoproteins). Chlorella contains mannose, arabinose and galactose amongst others. These help communication between cells, and your immune system to identify rogue cells.

A large number of Japanese studies has shown how both boost interferon and thus the white cells and particularly T-cells.

Chlorella seems to enhance levels of lactobacillus in the gut, another line of immune defence.

Both have excellent levels of beta-carotene (about ten times the level of carrots), organic iron and vitamins D and K. In chlorella, B vitamin levels are excellent, especially B-12, although folate levels are low.

Chlorella helps in detox diets since it can bind heavy metals and some pesticides.

The interesting development, though, is in the use of such chlorophyll-rich algae as agents in photodynamic therapy. Russian work shows that the chlorophyll, which produces oxygen when light is shone on it, can destroy cancer cells and US research (Waladkami, Clemens, 1990) has shown how important green vegetables and phytochemicals are in the restriction of cancer development.

There is an increasing body of opinion that chlorophyll (which has a similar molecular structure to haemoglobin) can circulate in the bloodstream and even help to oxygenate (and kill off) cancer cells. Eating your greens clearly pays off!

(xi) Herbs and other natural compounds

As animals in the wild we would take exercise prolifically and always be slightly hungry, both factors that help prevent cancer as we have seen. We would also have grazed – we would have had a vast number of foods we know were edible and by mixing our diet across this wide range we were more likely to have seen off cancer in its various stages.

The latter is an important point because, of course, cancer is a multi-step disease. There may be toxic build-up, a damaging step, multiplication of cancer cells, the supply of a blood system so the tumour can grow, then metastatic spread.

Nature could cope, it gave us herbs and other natural compounds like astragalus, bee propolis, anthocyanins (like the purple of beetroot and cherries), bromelain in pineapple, resveratrol in grapes and red wine, proanthocyanidis (like grape seed extract), polysaccharides (in mother's milk, leeks and garlic), plus a wealth of active ingredients in herbs like burdock, sheep sorrel, emodin, ginseng, feverfew, limonene, curcumin and flaxseed.

All of these can be dubbed 'antioxidants' or immune system boosters but not all work in the same way, each defending us against steps in the total cancer process. John Boik of the MD Anderson Cancer Institute in Houston, Texas, published a brilliant book in March 2001 looking in detail at how all of these work, and arguing that you needed to build a complete anti-cancer programme from all of them. The book has over 4000 detailed references and is called *Natural Compounds in Cancer Therapy*. His website is www.ompress.com. Your doctor may be concerned that some of these natural compounds may react with his prescribed drugs, but if you show him the book he can never deny that these natural compounds work. More information is available in the Third Edition of *Everything You Need to Know to Help you Beat Cancer*.

Overall

There is no doubt, if you want to beat cancer, that you cannot expect there to be a single magic pill. By now you should be building up a 'total picture', one where sodium and dairy are best avoided and potassium and magnesium foods given priority. Where weight control, exercise, and toxin-free air, water and foods are at a premium. And where vitamin supplements are imperative if you lead a hectic life, whilst the kitchen needs to be the home of garlic, fish oils, nuts and seeds, watercress and beetroot, olive oil and turmeric, red peppers and red clover, onions and oranges, acidophilus and apples.

The list brings new meaning to the phrase, 'a little of everything'.

CHAPTER 19

COOKING AND EATING TIPS

Although many books extol the benefits of raw food, others believe juicing helps to break up cellular structures and release minerals and enzymes. Some believe lightly cooking, even blanching, helps digestion and absorption.

Certainly the ideal is raw or lightly cooked, including steamed. Too many cooks wash the vitamins away with the boiled water.

Roasting is the next best route providing that little, if any, fat is used, and items are slow roasted with oven temperature ideally below 120°C, especially for potatoes (see acrylamides earlier). Boiled potatoes show no evidence of acrylamides.

Wood or coal barbecues are no-go areas. Smoke and flames burn the meat and increase levels of highly carcinogenic nitrosamines.

Fried food is linked to higher rates of hormonally driven cancers in women, and men who eat fried food regularly have a three-fold increase in cancer. Who needs the fats and oils, the insulin and oestrogen surges and the dangerous free-radicals?

Microwaves polarise general opinion but not mine! In one study, Kirlian photography (which shows the energetic forces naturally occurring around a body or a plant) showed a strong field around broccoli both in its raw state, and after steaming. But absolutely no energetic aura after just one second in a microwave. Every atom in every molecule in your food has electrons spinning in specific defined ways. In a microwave the atoms are energised to heat the food and it is absolutely impossible to expect all the electrons to be in the places they should have been when you turn off the microwave. You are eating irradiated, genetically modified food. William Kopp studies German and Russian papers on the subject and concluded that microwaved food is nutritionally deficient, and increases the number of cancerous cells circulating in the bloodstream. Beware, some restaurant chains only serve microwaved foods. Many restaurants use microwaves to defrost food.

Stews are actually full of nourishment. They are slow-cooked and the temperature is lower than would allow nitrosamines or acrylamides to form. The problem is fat levels.

'Woked food' is excellent, providing the oil is kept to a minimum, as it is in Asia. (In Asia water and oyster or fish sauce are actually used, not oil.) Vegetables are served crisper and retain higher nourishment values.

Learn to eat properly – a summary

- EAT FRESH, QUALITY, LIVING FOOD.
- If vegetables are eaten raw at the start of a meal (e.g. crudités, or raw vegetables with some dips), up to 40 per cent more vitamins and minerals are absorbed.
- Consumption of water before, during or at the end the meal should be avoided. Excess water merely dilutes the digestive enzymes and prevents them from working fully. Drink copious amounts of water but at least one and a half hours either side of a meal.
- Eat slowly and focus on the food. Reading, working or watching TV can cause a whole range of emotions and stress to alter your hormone balance and prevent the perfect uptake of vitamins and minerals.
- Chew thoroughly. This releases an enzyme in the saliva called ptyalin which is crucial to the proper digestion of carbohydrates.
- Try and eat four to six small meals per day to even out and maintain your blood sugar levels, and put less strain on your digestive tract, endocrine system and your pancreas.
- Eat less than you need and don't fill up on empty calories. Calorie restriction increases longevity through insulin and oestrogen limitation and stimulates human growth hormone production, which mops up free radicals and makes you leaner and fitter.
- **Do not eat carbohydrate and protein at the same time.** In the wild, our natural environment saw us find tubers and eat them, or gorge at a fruit tree, or capture an animal. We didn't take them all back to the cave and eat them on the same plate. Your digestive system is not designed for this total simultaneous consumption.

The carbohydrate and ptyalin mixture passes to the stomach where it needs an alkaline environment for maximum efficiency. Carbohydrate on its own clears the stomach in about one hour.

Protein on the other hand passes to the stomach where it meets its digestive enzyme pepsin and this requires an acid environment. Protein on its own can be digested in about one and a half hours.

But mix the two and the stomach doesn't know whether to be alkaline or acid, with the result that the food is improperly digested and takes up to eight hours to pass through. This results in inefficiency throughout the intestinal system. It is also further hampered in the over 50s who anyway produce less acid.

It is particularly important to people over 50 that they avoid mixing protein and carbohydrate on the same fork! Levels of acid in the stomach can anyway decline by 30 per cent after 50 making digestion and absorption of key vitamins a problem.

- If you believe you may have yeasts, fruit should always be consumed first, at the start of the meal and on an empty stomach, if at all. Otherwise it can sit on top of a meal and ferment. People on anti-yeast diets need to avoid this complication as the fermentation aids the growth of yeasts. Very sweet fruits are also to be avoided in this scenario. For healthy people without a yeast problem fruits may be eaten at any time.
- Vegetables, pulses and oats, for example, contain soluble fibre. This is essential to the alimentary canal where it dissolves, transports and helps excrete toxins and excess hormones. Organic, whole, brown rice should be eaten regularly as it is particularly good at cleansing your system.
- Green tea (especially decaffeinated) is a strong antioxidant and helps to balance any acidity in the food you have eaten. Red wine has similar benefits as we saw earlier.

SECTION C

THE 'ANTI-CANCER' DIET

INTRODUCTION

"The secret of success is consistency of purpose".
(Benjamin Disraeli)

By now you will have seen that a true cornucopia of food can be wonderful for you. A truly healthy diet is not one where food consumption is reduced to boredom or burden.

The problem with many diets is that they are so limiting, people tire of them. With The Tree of Life, *you are not likely to. There is so much you can eat, providing you add in the 'goodies'.*

If there is one restriction it is simply this. Be consistent. Stick at it, and you will be healthy and beat cancer. All things are possible in God's world.

CHAPTER 20

THE PLAN

Consistency of findings – a summary

It is interesting to note that whether the study is of Asian or French diets, glycoprotein foods rich in B-17 or potassium, the same foods come up time and time again as positive additions to our health.

For example, brown rice, garlic, watercress, sprouting seeds, radishes, pears, apples.

For example, yams are not just a good source of B-17, they produce alkaline-ash and are a precursor of DHEA, a hormone that helps mop up free radicals.

For example, almonds can provide analgesic effects, B-17 and good levels of calcium.

For example, sunflower seeds give you fibre, vitamin E and selenium.

But there are some foods which you leave out of your diet at your peril. For example:

- Fish – deep-sea caught fish is best because of fears of toxins in coastal waters. The best sources of omega 3 are salmon, herring, mackerel, sardines, and anchovies.
- Olive oil, walnut oil, flaxseed oil, nuts and seeds. Monounsaturated fats and oils protect by binding to free radicals. Nuts like almonds, walnuts and pecans contain a variety of nutrients from selenium to salicylin and fibre to B-17 and vitamin E.
- Garlic has a number of proven anti-cancer benefits especially when eaten fresh and raw.
- Ginger is another good anti-cancer agent, as are many natural herbs and spices like turmeric, linked to lower risk of colon cancer.
- Pulses, from lentils to chickpeas, and kidney to soya beans provide plant protein and protective phytoestrogens.
- Whole grains are important to a good diet; full of nutrients they release their energy slowly and so do not cause pancre-

atic stress and hormonal rushes. Oats, barley, buckwheat and millet, if unrefined, provide excellent sources of nourishment like B vitamins, E vitamins, glycoproteins and B-17.

- Crucial to your health is a diet rich in vegetables and fruit – the foliage of our tree of life. We cannot stress enough, FRESH IS BEST. Tomatoes, lightly cooked; red or yellow peppers, apples, apricots, radishes, cruciferous vegetables and broccoli, leeks and onions, etc, etc, etc.

The enemies of the diet

Dairy, farmed fish and meat, all processed foods and preservatives, all fried foods, fast foods, dried meats (pepperoni, bacon), frankfurters, sugar, salt, fizzy soft drinks, processed fruit juices, chips, crisps, biscuits, crispbreads and branded breakfast cereals (apart from muesli); caffeine, sweeteners (saccharine and aspartame) and all refined flour and rice products (pizzas, pasta, bread, jasmine rice, etc).

Meal making tips

- As we have said from the start this is not a diet of omission (apart from dairy and salt!!).
- A piece of meat can be eaten, but why not make it organic, why not add grilled tomatoes stuffed with garlic and parsley, or ratatouille from red peppers, tomatoes, onions, garlic and courgettes; or lentils stewed in red wine with onions, garlic and herbs?
- Don't eat a carbohydrate unless it is whole.
- Drink a glass of cabernet sauvignon (red wine), but only with your meal.
- Eat fish, use saffron to flavour it, or turmeric with the vegetables.
- Eat more salads with a variety of leaves, or only made from herbs, adding walnut or olive oil.
- Buy a wok and cook in oyster sauce or a little water. Cook chicken with lemongrass or slow boil it in coconut milk.
- Make your own breakfast muesli from whole grains, dried fruits, organic sunflower seeds, pumpkin seeds, crushed pecan nuts and a few psyllium seeds. Put out your snack bowl of seeds and nuts.
- Start your own vegetable garden: perpetual spinach, tomatoes in pots, green beans and cabbage. Plant an apple and a pear tree, keep a chicken or two.
- Have a herb garden – you can even do this in pots on your patio.
- Find a supplier of organic fruit and vegetables and a good supplier of meat and fish.
- Make your own bread without refined wheat, sugar or salt.
- Make your own juices using nourishing vegetables and fruit like carrots, ginger, and apples.
- Sprout your own seeds. Use mung beans or broccoli seeds in the bottom of a jar with a covering of water. They are full of anti-cancer agents.
- Make your own nourishing soups.
- Try a detox.

Be inspired. There is so much you can do.

The shopping trolley

The best way to plan your healthy diet is to prevent yourself being weak-willed. Pre-plan and only bring healthy foods into your home. *"It is not the mountains we conquer, but ourselves"*, according to Sir Edmund Hillary. Sometimes we just need a little help towards that self-discipline. Here is a look at what your shopping trolley can contain:

Make these your essentials:

FRUITS AND VEGETABLES

(Grow your own or buy organic as fresh as possible.)

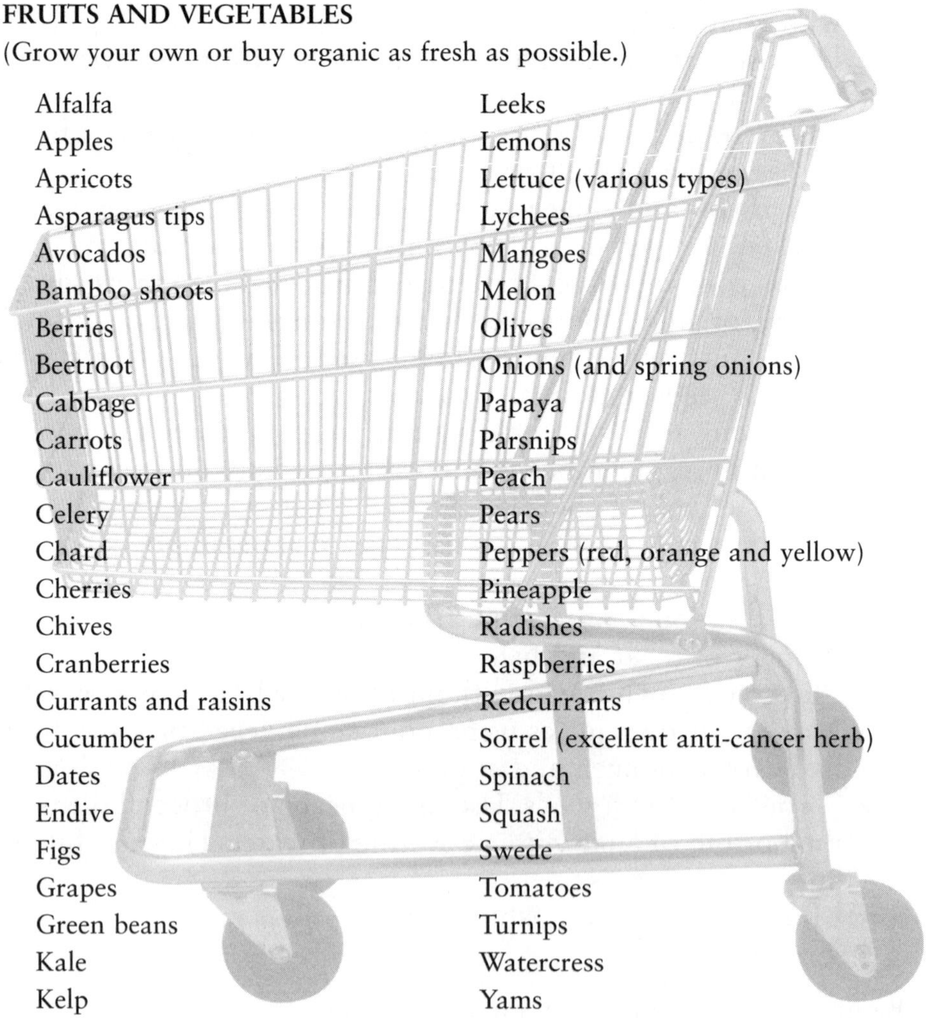

- Alfalfa
- Apples
- Apricots
- Asparagus tips
- Avocados
- Bamboo shoots
- Berries
- Beetroot
- Cabbage
- Carrots
- Cauliflower
- Celery
- Chard
- Cherries
- Chives
- Cranberries
- Currants and raisins
- Cucumber
- Dates
- Endive
- Figs
- Grapes
- Green beans
- Kale
- Kelp
- Leeks
- Lemons
- Lettuce (various types)
- Lychees
- Mangoes
- Melon
- Olives
- Onions (and spring onions)
- Papaya
- Parsnips
- Peach
- Pears
- Peppers (red, orange and yellow)
- Pineapple
- Radishes
- Raspberries
- Redcurrants
- Sorrel (excellent anti-cancer herb)
- Spinach
- Squash
- Swede
- Tomatoes
- Turnips
- Watercress
- Yams

PULSES
Broad beans
Butter beans
Chickpeas
Kidney beans
Lentils
Peas

WHOLE GRAINS
Barley
Buckwheat
Millet
Oats
Rye

NUTS
Almonds
Brazils
Cashews
Macadamia nuts
Pecans
Walnuts

SEEDS
Pumpkin
Sesame
Sunflower

OILS
Flaxseed oil
Olive oil
Walnut oil

HERBS / OTHER FLAVOURINGS
Basil
Coconut milk
Coriander
Fennel
Shoyu
Tamari
Tomato puree
Tomato sauces

SPICES
Chilli
Cinnamon
Nutmeg
Saffron
Turmeric

STAPLES
Aloe vera
Decaffeinated green teas
Fresh garlic and ginger
Herb teas
Honey
Limited amount of soya milk
Japanese mushrooms
Rice noodles
Whole brown rice

OTHER
Dried fruits, currants, raisins
Make your own fruit juices, muesli and soups
Oat bran
Psyllium seeds
Red wine (a glass of cabernet sauvignon per day – with meals)
Vegetarian hummus, pate, sausages, quorn

FISH / MEAT
Deep-sea caught fish
Organic chicken, turkey, pheasant, game, duck

We do not see the need to rule out meat, even the occasional piece of red meat. Organic would be best.

SUPPLEMENTS
Acidophilus
B-complex
Beta-carotene
Chlorella
CoQ10
Fish oils
Good liquid multivitamin and mineral supplement
Selenium
Vitamin E
Zinc

THE PROGRAMME

The aim is to keep it simple.

The target is 61 points per day. Real goodies should aim for 101 (especially those with cancer). Eat what you want but beat the target, everyday. Have fun.

DAILY PLATFORM

This is your start point each day. You can get a head start if you watch out for the following:

1) If you do 40 minutes exercise where your heart is continuously over 55 per cent of maximum heart rate (220 – your age x 55 per cent) + 15 points
2) If you filter your tap water with a reverse osmosis filter, and only drink with or cook in this water + 15 points
3) If you live outside a city centre and take exercise (e.g. yoga), or sport or energetic walks in the fresh air (not near main roads) + 5 points
4) If you are 2kgs underweight + 5 points
5) If you are 4kgs overweight – 3 points
6) If you are 10kgs overweight – 20 points
7) If you smoke at all (or work in/frequent a smokey place) – 20 points

POINTS FOR FOODS

All points have been assigned on a balance basis. For example baked beans have the benefits of tomato (sauce) and pulses, but the negatives of lots of sugar and salt and being canned.

Whole grain pasta is beneficial and achieves a positive score. Normal pasta is worthless.

FRESH IS BEST

Give yourself 3 points extra if you eat something organic, although strictly speaking, everything you eat should be organic.

This is meant to be a fun programme, so we have not assigned detailed weights or volumes.

The principle is that you can have your piece of lamb, if you really enjoy it, but put a tomato stuffed with garlic and parsley with it; perhaps some unrefined wild rice and lentils. This is how you pick up points and how you add in protective agents and eat to beat cancer.

It's not an ingredient but the totality of the meal that matters.

10 Points (1 serving e.g. large serving spoon)
FRESH, LOCALLY GROWN VEGETABLES AND FRUIT (LOW GI)

Alfalfa and sprouting seeds
Apples
Apricots
Asparagus tips
Berries
Beetroot
Cabbage
Cauliflower
Celery
Chard
Cherries
Chives
Cucumber
Endive
Garlic (1 clove raw)
Ginger
Green beans
Kale
Kelp
Leeks
Lettuce (various)
Olives
Onions
Parsnips
Peaches
Pears
Raspberries
Radishes
Redcurrants
Spring onions
Sorrel
Spinach
Squash
Swede
Tomatoes
Turnip
Watercress

FRESH NUTS

e.g. Almonds
Brazils
Cashews
Pecans
Macadamia nuts
Walnuts

SEEDS

Pumpkin
Sesame
Sunflower

PULSES

e.g. Broad beans
Butter beans
Chickpeas
Kidney beans
Lentils
Peas

DRINKS

1–2 glasses red wine especially Cabernet Sauvignon with meal (N.B. Alcohol outside meal score –5)

10 Points cont'd

OILS

Flaxseed oil
Linseed oil (linseeds)

FLESH

Deep-sea caught fish

CARBOHYDRATE AND GRAINS

Fresh boiled potato
Brown unrefined rice, wild rice
Oats, millet, barley, buckwheat
Unrefined grains

OTHER

Home-made muesli
Home-pressed fruit juices

5 Points

IMPORTED FRUITS AND VEGETABLES AND DRIED FRUITS

e.g. Avocados
Bamboo shoots
Bananas
Cranberries
Currants and raisins
Dates
Dried fruits
Figs
Grapes
Hot chillies
Lemons
Lychees
Mangoes
Melon
Papaya
Peppers
Satsumas
Yams

OTHERS

Aloe vera
Eggs – poached, boiled (free range and organic)
Garlic (cooked)

5 Points cont'd

Herbs – basil, fennel, coriander
Home-made bread (no salt, sugar – add seeds)
Honey
Hummus
Japanese mushrooms – e.g. Reishi, Maiitake, Cordyceps
Noni juice
Psyllium seeds
Spices – turmeric, chilli, cinnamon, nutmeg, saffron
Supermarket muesli, or non-baked cereals

FLESH

Locally caught fish

2 Points

OTHER

Baked potato
Canned fish
Canned fruit
Coconut milk
Green tea – 1 cup (decaffeinated)
Natural oat bran
Organic lean chicken, turkey, game (max 1 serving per day. Any further serving – 5 points.)
Potatoes (fresh) or mashed (no milk)
Quorn
Soups (chilled)
Soya and soy milk
Spices – chilli, cinnamon and nutmeg
Sweetcorn
Tomato sauces, puree (not ketchup)

1 Point

SUPPLEMENTS

Acidophilus – as directed on bottle (keep in 'fridge)
B complex – yeast-free, take as directed on bottle
Beta-carotene – 6 mgs, twice per day
Fish oils – 1000 mgs

1 Point cont'd

Vitamin C – 500 mgs, twice per day
Vitamin E – 400 IU
Zinc – 15 mgs
Selenium – 100 micrograms

N.B. If you take a good, ideally colloidal, vitamin and mineral supplement like Neway's Maximol you will not need to 'double up' with B complex, zinc or selenium. Score 3 points.

OTHER FRUITS

1 orange (max. per day)

0 Points

Bagels
Baked beans
Herb teas
Jams
Marmalade
Muesli bars, cereal bars
Organic bread
Organic meat, poultry, game
Processed fruit juices
Shoyu and tamari
Smoked fish
Soups
Stir-frying
Sunflower, safflower oils
Tomato ketchup
White wine
Wholemeal bread

–5 Points

Alcopops
Any processed food, ready meals (e.g. instant noodles, packaged soups), frozen meals
Beer, spirits, liqueurs
Biscuits

–5 Points cont'd

Bread, waffles – white or malted
Cakes
Chips
Chocolate snack products
Coffee
Crispbreads
Crisps, peanuts (salted)
Fizzy soft drinks
Mayonnaise
Pasta
Pizza
Processed breakfast cereals
Refined wheat, grains, sugar, rice
Rice cakes
Salt
Smoked meats
Sweeteners
Tea

–10 Points

Any dairy/milk product/yoghurts
Bacon, pepperoni, frankfurters, sausages, dried meats, pâté, rilletes
Barbecued food
Fast food (e.g. burgers, chicken portions, chips)
Fried foods
Hydrogenated vegetable oils
Margarines
Microwaved food
Pickled foods

CHAPTER 21
SOME INDICATIVE RECIPES

Introduction

As any one who has read dad's first book *Everything You Need to Know to Help You Beat Cancer* will know, I have a malignant brain tumour. I have had three operations in three years, two lots of radiotherapy and two short and unsuccessful rounds of chemotherapy.

All through this I have steadily improved my diet, taken supplements, taken up yoga and gone to the gym regularly. I've had a healer and tried all sorts of other helpful anti-cancer therapies. I can tell you that no one knows more about diets and cancer than me! Coming home from radiotherapy without an ounce of energy in your body, or having chemotherapy and feeling sick for days, or having no white cells and having to inject yourself to get some sort of immune system back; although I lost weight it was not as bad as it could have been.

I have also been surrounded by a wonderful family and exceptional friends, all of whom have helped pick me up when it mattered and made me laugh and given me fun and enjoyment. I met Dr Contreras and was interested that fun nights and sing-along sessions were actually a part of his cancer treatment programme at the Oasis of Hope. I'm not surprised. I've always tried to get on with my life, to focus on the future and to that end I have taken courses from photography to cookery.

I was going to write my own book on eating. I wanted the recipes to use ingredients you could buy from your normal supermarket (who has the energy to chase around for special, often exotic, ingredients after chemotherapy?). I wanted to develop nourishing meals to fight the weight loss and debilitation. And I wanted to suggest meals that could easily be taken out of the freezer on days when you are feeling terrible. Of course you don't have to have cancer to eat these dishes! They are just healthy, tasty and nourishing anyway.

Anyway, instead I decided to add these recipes to this second edition of *The Tree of Life*. I hope you enjoy them.

At least you know they have had patient approval – me!

Best wishes

Catherine

BREAKFAST

1. Homemade Muesli

Oats
Millet flakes
Pumpkin seeds
Sunflower seeds
Almonds
Cracked walnuts
Cashews

Create a large bowl or tin of your muesli so that there's no need to make it up every day. Then add dried apricots or peaches and a spoon of linseed before adding your rice or soya milk. Remember to buy organic, where possible.

* *The millet, almonds and cashews contain B-17, and the seeds vitamin E, omega 3 and selenium. High in fibre and slow release carbohydrate. You can add 5 or 6 bitter apricot kernels too if you want. Don't forget to take some acidophilus as well!*

2. Fruit Salad

Kiwis
Banana
Grapes
Pineapple
Papaya
Melon

This is a fantastic dish to make up in a huge bowl and then you can tuck into it throughout the day or serve as a fab pudding. Try any combination that you fancy!

* *Full of vitamin C and minerals like potassium.*

3. Citrus Salad

(Serves 4)

2 tbsp active manuka honey (New Zealand honey available from good health food shops)
120 ml freshly squeezed citrus juice (e.g. orange and grapefruit)
1 white grapefruit
1 pink grapefruit*
2 oranges
1 blood orange (or another pink grapefruit)
6–8 fresh dates, stoned and halved
Fresh mint leaves, thinly chopped

Mix the honey and citrus juice in a small saucepan, bring to the boil, then reduce heat and simmer for about 6 minutes or until slightly thickened. Peel the fruits, removing the white pith. Slice them crossways and remove the pips. Arrange the fruit in a serving bowl. Pour the hot syrup over and arrange the dates over the top. Sprinkle with mint. Serve within three hours of making.

* *Pink grapefruit is a good source of Lycopene, and Manuka honey is strongly anti-bacterial.*

4. Grilled Tomatoes on Toast

2 fresh tomatoes, sliced in half
4 slices of bread (wholemeal or granary)
A little parsley and watercress to serve

Again this is very simple. Place the tomato halves under a medium heat grill. Grill them until soft and slightly brown. Meanwhile toast the bread, ideally a granary or wholemeal to provide you with the most fibre. (This will help get your digestion moving after all the anti-sickness tablets have caused constipation.) Once the tomatoes are grilled simply place them on the toast and voila! Serve with parsley and watercress. Mushrooms make a tasty accompaniment.

Tip: Add a little fresh garlic for further cancer fighting agents.

* *Cooked tomatoes especially release their lycopene. Whole grain bread gives you plenty of B vitamins.*

5. Wake Up Smoothie

250 ml oat, soya or rice milk
15 ml oatbran
2 tsps peanut butter
Juice of ½ lemon or lime
1 banana
1 tsp honey

Blend all the ingredients together, pour into glasses and serve immediately.

* *Rich in B vitamins, protein, calcium, vitamin B6 and potassium.*

6. Egg and Spinach Scramble

2 eggs (organic free range)
A little soya milk
Freshly ground black pepper to taste
50 g baby spinach leaves*

Break the eggs into a bowl, whisk, adding a splash of soya milk and black pepper to taste. Using a small non-stick saucepan, slowly cook the eggs, whisking continually on a low heat. As the eggs begin to thicken add the spinach leaves and serve immediately.

* *Spinach is a good source of several antioxidants, including vitamins C and E. It provides useful amounts of folate, niacin and B6. Along with the eggs this would be good during radiotherapy.*

Eggs

Eggs are healthy – it's how you cook them that is usually the problem! Occasionally an egg for breakfast makes a nice change. Buy organic free range eggs only and these can be served poached with the above grilled tomatoes dish. Organic free range eggs will help your DNA during radiotherapy.

For breakfast, drink peppermint tea; or make your own lemon and fresh ginger – add a little honey to taste. Green tea is also very protective.

LUNCHES AND SNACK MEALS

7. Tomato and Red Pepper Soup

(Serves 4)

4 fresh tomatoes, skinned and finely chopped
400 g tin tomatoes
1 red pepper, deseeded and finely chopped
1 garlic clove, crushed
1 onion, finely chopped
Handful of fresh tarragon, chopped (or a teaspoon of dried)
Olive oil

Place 1 teaspoon (maximum) of olive oil in a large pan, slowly cook the onion and crushed garlic for about five minutes until they have softened. Add the fresh tomatoes and red pepper, fry for another couple of minutes then add the tin of tomatoes and 2 tins full of water*. Stir in the chopped tarragon saving a little to use as a garnish with and leave to simmer for 1 hour stirring occasionally.

Tip: This dish is highly nutritious with loads of antixodiants. If you're having chemotherapy, it's good to cook this the day before and keep it in the fridge so if you're tired you just have to re-heat it.

* *Reminder: Best to use reverse osmosis filtered water or still mineral water (glass bottled).*

8. Pumpkin Soup

"For those cold autumnal days and great for the kids at Halloween!"

(Serves 4)

1 carrot, sliced
1 medium potato, peeled and chopped
1 onion, chopped
700 g pumpkin flesh, chopped
600 ml vegetable stock (see recipe 19)
1 tbsp extra virgin olive oil
2.5 cm fresh ginger, peeled and grated
1 garlic clove, finely chopped
½ tsp grated nutmeg
½ tsp ground coriander
Freshly ground black pepper

Heat the olive oil in large pan, add the onion and saute for about 5 minutes or until translucent. Add the ginger, garlic, nutmeg and coriander, stir and cook for 1 minute. Add the vegetables and continue cooking for 5 minutes. Pour in the stock, bring to boil then simmer for 20 minutes or until the vegetables are tender. Take off the heat and allow to cool. Liquidise in a blender or food processor. Season to taste with freshly ground pepper. Serve hot.

Tip: You can always add a little more water or stock to make it a little thinner.

* *Pumpkin is rich in the phytonutrient alpha carotene, which also helps prevent cancer. Also rich in vitamin E, vitamin C and beta-carotene. Coriander and nutmeg are anti-bacterial and anti-yeast.*

9. Carrot and Coriander Soup

(Serves 4)

4 carrots, sliced or diced however you prefer!
1 onion, chopped
1 medium potato, sliced or diced
Handful of fresh coriander or a teaspoon of ground pepper
1.5 litres vegetable stock (see recipe 19)
Grated nutmeg
Olive oil

In a large pan, fry the onion in a little olive oil until soft. Add the carrots and continue for a few minutes. Next add the potato and vegetable stock, and finally stir in the coriander and half a teaspoon of grated nutmeg. Simmer for about an hour – until it is the consistency for you. I like to then put mine in a blender and serve it with a spoonful of low fat crème fraiche and a sprinkling of fresh coriander. Umm delicious!

Tip: Add some fresh garlic for extra taste.

"All win, win if you ask me!"

10. Spicy Parsnip Soup

(Serves 4)

225 gms parsnips, peeled and sliced
150 gms swede, peeled and diced
125 gms turnip, peeled and diced
1 onion, finely chopped
2 tbsp extra virgin olive oil
1 tsp ground cumin or turmeric
1 tsp ground coriander
A little freshly grated nutmeg
Freshly ground black pepper
600 ml vegetable stock (see recipe 19)

Heat the olive oil in a saucepan over a moderate heat, add the onion and saute for about 5 minutes or until it is translucent. Stir in the spices and continue to cook for about 1 minute, stirring continuously. Add the vegetables and stir to coat. Cook over a moderate heat in a covered pan for about 5 minutes. Add the stock, bring to the boil and simmer for about 15 minutes or until the vegetables are tender. Take off the heat and allow to cool. Liquidise in a blender or food processor. Season to taste with nutmeg and freshly ground pepper. Serve hot.

Tip: Soups are also great to keep for a while, use as starters at dinner parties and in general provide you with loads of tasty vegetables, or could be frozen in individual servings and used on the days when you just don't feel like cooking!

* *Parsnips, swede and turnip are all rich in 'perky potassium', and swede is a good source of vitamin C too. Cumin is a good anti-oxidant.*

11. Crudités served with Dips

"To make your crudités some suggestions of fab vegetables are:"

Carrots
Red pepper
Fennel*
Broccoli**
Celery
Small sweetcorns

These are all great vegetables but do add any of your own favourites. Best to cut enough for you on to a plate and consume raw.

Tip: Try different combinations and see what your favouites are. Always wash vegetables thoroughly and remember to buy organic.

* *Fennel is high in potassium and anti-fungal.*
** *Broccoli contains indole 3 carbinol which can fight cancer*

12. Hummus Dip

200 g tin chick peas (or dried, just remember to soak!)
80 ml extra virgin olive oil
3–4 tablespoons lemon juice
2 garlic cloves, crushed or finely chopped
1 tbsp cumin seeds, browned in a frying pan then crushed

This is so simple – in a large bowl crush the chickpeas and mix in the other ingredients – and season to your taste! How simple is that? This will also keep for a while too.

Tip: I love to serve this with hot crusty wholemeal bread.

* *Full of phytoestrogens.*

13. Tomato Salsa Dip

"For days when you are feeling a little Mexican!"

4 tomatoes
1 red chilli
1 garlic clove
1 green or red pepper (green gives different colour but in fairness you get more goodness from the red)
Handful of basil

Finely chop all the ingredients and mix together for a gorgeous and spicy hot dip! Very good for you.

Tip: If you have a blender, just put all the ingredients together and save yourself some time!

14. Yoghurt, Mint and Cucumber Dip

1/4 cucumber
150 ml/g natural soya yoghurt
Handful chopped fresh mint

Combine all the ingredients together in a blender to make a delicious dip.

Tip: This could also be a fab accompaniment to the fajitas for dinner!

15. Mixed Salad

Lettuce, any type (a combination of different ones is fab or you could use different herbs: thyme, coriander, baby spinach etc.)
Tomato
Sweetcorn (ideally taken from the corn and cooked, however, if you do not have time the tinned variety can be used but only if low in sugar and salt)
Red pepper
Cucumber
Fennel
Apple

Chop and cut the above in quantities that you prefer and then serve with a low fat dressing for a very balanced diet.

Tip: For a great vinaigrette dressing simply use the following:
Balsamic vinegar
1 garlic clove, crushed
Olive oil
The best combination I've ever tried is mixing the olive oil and vineger in a 3:1 mix however try it out and see what you prefer. Try whipping it up with a 1/4 to 1/2 a half teaspoon of wholegrain mustard.

16. Salad Niçoise

"A favourite of mine, a reminder of lovely days in the sun on beaches in the South of France."

Lettuce (though better to use a mixture of organic herb leaves and waterceress)
Tuna (best to buy a small tuna steak and grill it, or if from a can, in spring water)
Black olives**
Small new potatoes (although traditionally these are not included in the Mediterranean recipe)
Green beans
Red onions

French vinaigrette dressing: made of olive oil and red wine vinegar mixed in 3:1 proportions, and ½ tsp mustard. Place the ingredients in a lidded jar and give it a good shake! You can keep the dressing in the fridge for a week.

Steam the new potatoes and green beans until tender, then leave to cool. Prepare the tuna and cool. Prepare the vinaigrette (see above). Slice the red onions into fine rings. Arrange the salad leaves in a bowl and pour the vinaigrette over and toss it when you are just about to eat. Add the onions followed by the cooked tuna, cooked potatoes, green beans and top with roughly chopped black olives.

Tip: If you want to get more traditional still, add anchovies then chop some fresh pink garlic into the salad. This original Nice dish rarely had tuna but was made with anchovies and lots of garlic and olive oil – full of health.

* *Full of vitamins and omega 3*
** *Black olives are rich in monosaturated fats and vitamin E*

17. Banana and Cauliflower Salad

(Serves 4)

2 bananas
300 gms tiny cauliflower florets
55 gms cashew nuts, chopped
1 tsp cumin seeds
2 tbsp fresh thyme leaves
juice of 1/2 a lemon
1 tbsp olive oil
3 sharon fruit, peeled and cut into small pieces
4 tbsp fresh chives, cut
Fresh thyme to garnish

Steam the cauliflower florets for 1–2 minutes. Rinse under cold running filtered water. Leave to drain and cool. In a heavy duty frying pan, brown the nuts, cumin seeds and thyme leaves, tip into a bowl and leave to cool. Slice the bananas and put in a mixing bowl, add the lemon juice to coat. Add the cauliflower florets and nut mixture and olive oil. Toss gently to mix. Add the sharon fruit and chives and fold in. Cover and leave to marinate for 30 minutes. Spoon the salad into serving dish and garnish with fresh thyme.

Tip: This unusual salad uses both sweet and sharp fruit with nuts to add colour and interest to the cauliflower florets. Can be served with a green salad or on its own.

"Sounds wacky, but absolutely delicious!"

18. Risotto

Basic recipe:

Araborio rice
1.5 litres of vegetable stock (see recipe 19)
1 tsp of mixed herbs
Parmesan (can be omitted if not eating dairy)

Place the rice and mixed herbs in a large pan and start to add the stock in ladles full at a time. Only add more stock once the previous amount has been absorbed. Once all the stock has been absorbed, taste. If a little hard then add a few more ladles of water until soft. Once cooked, throw in your parmesan and serve immediately.

* *This recipe should be used as a base for recipes 20 and 21, but can also be made using shitake mushrooms for high glycoprotein levels.*

19. Vegetable Stock

To make 600ml (1 pint)

900 ml water
2 onions
2 carrots
2 celery sticks
1 leek
Fresh thyme and/or parsley

Slice all the vegetables and herbs and put into large pan. Bring to the boil and simmer gently for about 1 hour. Leave to cool. Strain and use.

20. Broccoli, Pea and Chicken Risotto

(Serves 4)

1 basic risotto recipe (see recipe 18)
1 medium broccoli floret, chopped
2 tbsp peas (can use frozen)
200 g chicken breast, finely chopped
1 medium onion, finely sliced
1 garlic clove, crushed
Olive oil
Pinch of mixed herbs

In a large pan heat a little olive oil and slowly soften the onion and garlic. Then add the chicken. Once browned add the rice, peas, broccoli and mixed herbs and cook as in the basic recipe.

21. Sweetcorn, Broccoli and Goat's Cheese Risotto

1 basic risotto recipe (see recipe 18)
2 tbsp sweetcorn (can be frozen, but must be organic)
1 medium broccoli floret, chopped
100 g soft goat's cheese

Add the rice, sweetcorn and broccoli to a large pan and cook as in the basic recipe. When finally cooked instead of adding the parmesan, stir in the goat's cheese until it has melted and serve immediately.

22. Spaghetti Arboreta

350 g spaghetti (corn or rice spaghetti preferably)
1 medium onion
1 garlic clove
400 g tin tomatoes
1 red pepper, finely chopped
1 red chilli, seeds removed, then finely chopped
Handful of basil, ripped

In a large pan bring the water to the boil and add the spaghetti, boil according to the instructions on the packet.

In another pan soften the onion, garlic and chilli for about five minutes then add the red pepper and cook for another couple of minutes. Then add the tinned tomatoes and the ripped basil. Once simmering, drain your spaghetti and serve with the sauce on top.

Tip: Always warm the serving bowl and plates before serving as spaghetti cools very quickly.

23. Tuna and Bean Salad

(Serves 4)

400 gms tuna steak
4 tbsp extra virgin olive oil
400 g can cannellini beans, drained and rinsed
1 small red onion, thinly sliced
2 red peppers, seeded and thinly sliced
½ cucumber, diced
100 g watercress
1 tbsp lemon juice
1 garlic clove, finely chopped
1 tbsp Dijon mustard
Freshly ground black pepper
Lemon wedges to serve

Brush the tuna on both sides with a little olive oil and season on both sides with the freshly ground pepper. In a heavy frying pan seal the tuna on both sides and cook gently to prevent over-cooking as it can become too dry. The tuna should be light pink in the centre. Remove tuna and leave to rest. Mix together the remaining oil, lemon juice, garlic and mustard. Season with black pepper and additional lemon juice to taste if required. Put the beans, onion, peppers and cucumber in a salad bowl. Add the watercress and then most of the dressing (keeping a little to spoon over the fish at the end) and toss to mix. Cut the tuna into 1 cm thick slices. Arrange on top of the salad and spoon the remaining dressing on the top. Serve with lemon wedges.

Tip: Replace tuna with chicken by using organic, skinless, boneless chicken breast fillet. Cook in pan for about 20 minutes or until chicken thoroughly cooked through. Turn it frequently to avoid sticking. Leave to cool and serve as per tuna above.

* *Watercress provides good levels of vitamins and minerals including vitamin B-17, C and E plus B vitamins folate, niacin and vitamin B2. Canned beans are a good source of iron, but rinse them before use.*

24. Khao Tom Kai
(Chicken, Coriander and Garlic Breakfast Bowl)

(Serves 2 – for breakfast or as a snack)

2 chicken breasts, boned and skinned
1 tbsp Thai fish sauce (nam pla)
2 tbsps chopped fresh spring onion
2 tbsps fresh ginger, peeled and cut into the size of matchsticks (plus a few more for garnish)
2 tbsps chopped fresh coriander leaves
1 tsp ground black pepper
2 tbsps chopped fresh garlic
Half cup of brown rice

Cook the rice in a pan. Slice the chicken thinly against the grain and chop until small. Add the chicken and the garlic to the pan and wait until the chicken is cooked. Then add the ginger. Add in the Thai fish sauce (nam pla), black pepper and chopped fresh coriander leaves, plus more of the ginger matchsticks to garnish and serve.

Tip: You eat this with any excess boiled water still in the bowl. This dish is healthy and full of energy; an amazing breakfast although you can enjoy your meal any time in the morning, as it is not heavy and yet very tasty.

* *Full of vitamins and anti-yeast garlic and ginger.*

25. Laab Gai
(Chicken, Coriander, Garlic and Chilli)

(Serves 2 – for lunch)

2 chicken breasts, boned, skinned and chopped
2 tbsps Thai fish sauce (nam pla)
2 tbsps mint, chopped
2 tbsps coriander leaves, chopped
2 tbsps fresh garlic, chopped
2 tbsps fresh spring onion, chopped
2 tbsps lemon juice
1 tbsp dried red chillies, crushed
2 tbsps sticky rice, dry fried for 8–10 mins, then pounded
2 kaffir lime leaves, finely sliced
6 fresh or soya green beans
6 large lettuce leaves
2.5 cm cucumber, chopped

Boil the chicken in a small pan of water until cooked. Mix in the mint, spring onion, coriander leaves, and then the garlic. Add the lemon juice, and Thai fish sauce (nam pla) plus the rice, lime leaves and the red chillies and mix everything together. You may add more spring onions to garnish. To serve place 3 large lettuce leaves on a plate and put the chopped cucumber, 3 green beans and spring onions on top. Pour the laab gai next to it.

Tip: This traditional Thai dish from the north east of Thailand is a delicious, tasty meal. It is used as a lunch or dinner and is yummy! You may also have a bowl of steamed brown rice to accompany it.

DINNER

26. Dover Sole with Lemon

(Serves 2)

1 lemon, grate and juice so that you have the zest and juice
1 Dover sole (ask your fishmonger to remove all the bones or you can buy fillets)

This is so simple, just place under a medium heat grill or in a frying pan on the lowest heat and cook. I like to marinate mine with a little of the lemon zest and juice but, as always, that's up to your taste.

Season and serve with brown rice and vegetables such as minted peas or broccoli.

27. Salmon Parcels

(Serves 4)

4 salmon steaks (fresh, not farmed and must be organic)
1 onion, sliced into four for the steaks to sit on
150 g black olives, stones removed and roughly chopped
2 lemons and/or limes
1 tbsp white wine
Sprigs of dill

Preheat oven to 190°C. On a piece of tin foil lay a slice of onion, then the salmon steak. Coat with a sprinkling of lime or lemon juice and place dill sprigs on top. Sprinkle olives over the top and add a tablespoon of white wine. Encase the package and place in the oven for 30 minutes.

* *Fish is great for providing omega 3 oils. In plain English, brain food and anti-cancer food!*

28. Roast Chicken

"This is so easy and absolutely delicious – even if I do say so myself!"

(Serves 4)

1 medium chicken
4 garlic cloves, sliced
2 lemons, limes or oranges, zest and juice then keep skins and some juice as stuffing
Herbs (your preference but ideally either fresh thyme or rosemary)

Slice the garlic, add the fruit zest and herbs. Place this mixture under the chicken skin (both breast and legs). To stuff the bird, use the fruit skins, juice and any remaining garlic, fruit zest and herb mixture. Cook the chicken at 180°C for 30 minutes per 450g (1lb) plus an extra 30 minutes. Ensure the chicken is thoroughly cooked by inserting a thin knife or skewer into the bird meat – the juices should run clear.

Tip: If you like onion gravy stand the chicken on a couple of thick slices of onion. You can then use it with the chicken juices to make a gravy.

Also, with it try **Lentils and Red Onions**

Drop a teaspoon of olive oil into a saucepan and add two chopped garlic cloves, then one chopped red onion. When this is just softening after about two minutes, add in a cup of lentils (black Le Puy are best) and quickly mix into the oil. Then add three to four cups of water, and bring to the boil and simmer for about 15–20 minutes. Very, very healthy and full of protective phytoestrogens. Serve with a few small carrots and some broad beans or broccoli.

29. Chicken in Coconut Milk

(Serves 4)

4 chicken breasts, skin removed
2 cloves of garlic, crushed or chopped
2 cm ginger, grated
Lemongrass, crushed
Coriander, chopped
400 ml tin of coconut milk

Mix the garlic, ginger and lemongrass. Make a pocket along the side of your chicken and stuff with this mixture. Seal the pocket with either a cocktail stick or tie with string. You can either leave this to marinate for an hour or, if in a rush, you can cook immediately. Brown the chicken and place in an ovenproof dish. Coat the chicken with coriander and cover with coconut milk. Cook at 180°C for 30–45 minutes until chicken is thoroughly cooked through. Remember to remove the cocktail stick or string before serving!

* *Lemongrass has 100 times the antioxidant power of beta-carotene. Ginger, like garlic, is an excellent anti-cancer agent as well as being anti-fungal.*

30. Chicken with Spices

"This is great to make loads of so that on those days when you feel a little rough you can always defrost some and have it in a salad or sandwich."

8 chicken legs and thighs (skin on)

Sauce:
1½ tbsps olive oil
1 tsp cumin seeds
½ tsp cardamom pods
1 red chilli, finely chopped
1 red pepper, finely chopped
1 onion, finely chopped
150 ml natural soya yogurt
50 ml water

Marinade:
2 tsps turmeric
2 garlic cloves, crushed
2 cm ginger, grated

Mix the marinade ingredients together, coat the chicken and leave to marinate for at least an hour. Meanwhile brown the cardamom pods and cumin seeds in a frying pan then crush with the chilli. Fry the onion in a little olive oil; when soft, add the red pepper and fry for a minute, then add in the chilli, cardamom and cumin and continue to cook for a couple of minutes. Remove from heat and combine with the yogurt and water.

Brown the marinated chicken and place in a baking dish. Cover the chicken with the sauce mixture and cook, covered, at 185°C for 30 minutes. At this point remove the cover, stir and cook for a further 15 minutes or until chicken is thoroughly cooked through.

Tip: To make it a little sweeter use a red onion

* *Onions, garlic, chilli and cumin are all great helpers in your fight against cancer.*

31. Fajitas

(Serves 4)

1 onion, chopped
2 peppers (red and/or green, yellow or orange), sliced
2 garlic cloves, crushed
1 cm ginger, grated
4 chicken breasts, sliced length ways for nice long strips!
1 red chilli, finely chopped (can omit if you don't like things very spicy, but I dare you to try!)
Wholemeal flat bread or pitta bread
Olive oil

Saute the onion, garlic and ginger in olive oil until softened, stirring continuously. Add the sliced chicken, peppers and chilli. Continue to stir until the chicken is thoroughly cooked through. Serve immediately in flat bread or pitta bread.

Tip: Serve with tomato salsa (recipe 13) or hummus (recipe 12) and mixed leaves or lettuce.

32. Chicken Parcels with Fennel

"I found these parcels fab to make before chemo and then I could easily defrost one on days when I was too tired to cook. Make sure you defrost thoroughly before cooking."

(Serves 2)

2 chicken breasts, boned and skinless
1 fennel bulb, sliced (keep the feathers for garnishing)
1 large tomato, thickly sliced
2 sprigs of rosemary
100 g of black olives, stones removed and roughly chopped
Extra virgin olive oil

In a frying pan slowly fry the fennel with a little olive oil, until it has softened and turned slightly brown. Divide the fennel and juices in half and place on two large pieces of tin foil. Onto the fennel add a large slice of tomato, a sprig of rosemary, the chicken breast and top with the olives. Seal the foil to make a parcel and bake for approximately 30 minutes at 180°C or until chicken is thoroughly cooked.

33. Lamb Shanks

"This is fab as a casserole dish – one you can just chuck together and then ignore for an hour!"

(Serves 4)

4–6 lamb shanks
2 garlic cloves, sliced
Handful of fresh rosemary
1 onion, finely chopped
400 ml tin of tomatoes
100 g sun dried tomatoes, chopped

Insert a small knife deep into the shank at various places and push in some garlic and rosemary. In a frying pan add a little olive oil and soften the onions. Put the lamb shanks, softened onion, sun dried tomatoes and the tinned tomatoes in an oven-proof dish. Cover and bake for about one hour on a low heat (180°C). Serve with brown whole rice, lentils and a grilled tomato with chopped garlic on top.

34. Chilli Con Carne

"This was one of my favourites to cook and save in separate portions for days when I just didn't have the energy to cook. You can always use quorn if you think you should avoid meat. If served with a baked potato (oven baked, never microwaved), it is easy to bring out of the freezer and is so nourishing! Always a bonus ... hee hee!

500 g low fat organic mince
1 onion (red if you fancy it), chopped
2 garlic cloves, crushed
2 cm ginger, grated
1 red chilli, finely chopped
1 tsp cumin powder
1–2 tsps of chilli powder (go on how daring are you!)
1 red pepper
2 400 ml tins tomatoes
2 400 ml tins red kidney beans
Serve with whole brown or basmati rice, or baked potato

In a large pan, add a little olive oil and soften the onions, garlic and ginger. Once softened, add in the cumin, chilli powder and red chilli, and fry for a minute or two then add the mince. Fry all until browned and drain off any excess fat, then add the red pepper and tinned tomatoes. Cook for at least an hour on a low heat so that all the spices are absorbed. In the last half hour stir in the red kidney beans.

Tip: I love this dish on top of a split baked potato – always a great pick me up and great to warm the body too!

As we have stated throughout, a little meat is no bad thing provided you accompany it with foods that can neutralise the fats like lycopene, olive oil and garlic.

35. Vegetarian Curried Lentil and Vegetable Pilaf

(Serves 4)

400 ml coconut milk
600 ml vegetable stock (recipe 19)
2 tbsp olive oil
1½ tsp cumin seeds
2 tsp ground coriander
2.5 cm fresh ginger, grated
1 garlic clove, crushed
½ tsp cayenne pepper
200 gms brown rice
200 gms red lentils
500 gms prepared and chopped mixed vegetables, e.g. carrots, broccoli, green beans and cauliflower
Fresh ground black pepper
Chopped fresh coriander or parsley to garnish

Heat the oil in a lidded pan and add the cumin seeds and stir until they sizzle. Stir in the coriander, ginger, garlic and cayenne pepper, and stir fry for about a minute. Stir in the rice, lentils and vegetables, then pour in the stock and coconut milk, mix together. Bring to the boil, reduce the heat, then cover and simmer for about 20 minutes, or until the rice and lentils are tender and the liquid has been absorbed. Add the freshly ground black pepper to season. Sprinkle with chopped coriander or parsley.

Tip: Can be served with sliced bananas with lime juice squeezed over, and a little grated lime zest to garnish.

36. Baked Onions

Serve on their own or with roast chicken (see recipe 28)

(Serves 4)

8 medium onions
Freshly ground black pepper
50 g soya butter
2 tbsp chopped parsley

Wash the onions in their skins, removing as much grit as possible and then dry them well. Line a baking tin with foil to prevent the onions sticking to the tin. Put in the onions and bake in a preheated oven (180°C) for 2–3 hours until tender when pierced with a skewer. Sprinkle with freshly ground black pepper and put a knob of soya butter on each. If you like you can flavour the soya butter with cinnamon and cayenne pepper. Garnish with parsley and serve.

SWEET THINGS AND PUDDINGS

37. Blueberry and Raspberry Mousse

(Serves 4)

225 g fresh raspberries
125 g fresh blueberries
300 g silken tofu
2 tbsp honey
Mint leaves to garnish

Place the fruit in a blender with the tofu and honey. Blend until smooth, put into four individual dishes. Chill and serve.

* *Blueberries and raspberries are rich in vitamin C and ellagic acid. Blueberries are rich in phytonutrients and high in antioxidants. The tofu is a good source of protein.*

38. Fresh Fruit Fondue

Fruit
Select a good variety of fresh fruits e.g. strawberries, raspberries, cherries (with stalks) – keep them whole, plus pineapple and bananas chopped into chunks.

Place on a baking sheet and put into the freezer for about 1 hour – to chill, not freeze!

Fondue
Sugar free carob drops (from good health food shops)
2 tbsp maple syrup
2 tsp vanilla essence
Melt in a 'bain-marie' (double saucepan) or fondue.

Serve to guests the hot fondue with the tray of fruit. Dip fruits on fondue forks into the warm mixture. The chilled fruits will set the fondue around them – warm on the outside and chilled inside.

Delicious and an easy dessert for guests to 'cook' themselves!

39. Plum and Almond Parcels

(Serves 4)

8 purple plums*
125 g fresh orange juice
2 tsps honey
2 tsps flaked almonds, crushed
Few drops of almond essence

Cut the plums in half and remove the stones, then place in a shallow baking dish. Pour orange juice and almond essence over the plums, trickle with honey and top with almonds. Cover with tin foil and bake in a low oven (180°C) for 30 minutes or until tender. Serve warm or chilled with soya cream.

* *Plums are a good source of fibre and have good antioxidant benefits. They contain hydroxycinnamic acid which is associated with a reduced risk of colon cancer.*

40. Baked Apples

(Serves 4)

4 large cooking apples, preferably Bramleys

Choose one of the following fillings:

- 1 large banana, finely chopped and mixed with 1/2 tsp cinnammon
- 4 oz dried apricots, chopped with manuka honey
- 4 oz dried dates, chopped with 2 oz of nuts and the juice of a lemon

Core the apples and score the skin round the middle of each. Stand them in a deep dish. Fill the cavities with your chosen filling. Bake in a pre-heated oven (180°C), for about 1 hour. Serve hot or cold.

Tip: For an alternative try baked pears and reduce the cooking time accordingly.

SMOOTHIES AND SHAKES

REMEMBER TO ADD THE INGREDIENTS BEGINNING WITH LIQUIDS AND ENDING WITH SOLIDS

41. Mango, Melon and Ginger Shake

1 mango, peeled and stoned then cut into chunks*
2 cm fresh ginger, grated
80 g cantaloupe melon, cubed
250 ml soya milk
Handful of crushed ice

Put mango, melon, ice and soya milk into a blender, add the ginger, blend and serve immediately.

* *Mango is rich in beta-carotene, magnesium and vitamin C. Also potassium and calcium.*

42. Carrot, Apple, Beetroot and Celery Smoothie

(Makes 2 glasses)

2 carrots
1 apple
1/4 beetroot
2 celery sticks

Blend all the ingredients together, pour into glasses and serve immediately.

* *Rich in beta-carotene, vitamin C, potassium and antioxidant nutrients.*

43. Traffic Light Smoothie

(Makes 2 glasses)

2 carrots
1 red pepper
1 yellow pepper

Blend all the ingredients together, pour into glasses and serve immediately.

* *Carrots and peppers are rich in beta-carotene – a major plank of the Gerson Therapy. Also lots of vitamin C.*

APPENDICES

APPENDIX I

Reverse osmosis water filters

Water Filtration

A brief summary of some of the more common approaches:

1. **Bottled and spring water**: the water quality is highly variable between one source and another. Bottled waters may become contaminated by synthetic oestrogens in plastic bottles if stored for some time. Some bottlers treat their water with ozone, deionisation, carbon or micron filtration. Some bottled waters are also high in sodium. People very seldom use bottled water to cook with. However, some spring waters have healing properties and this might be associated with the unique structure of these waters. Maximum benefit is to be had by drinking these waters at source.
2. **Carbon filters**. There are many different forms of carbon or charcoal filter. The simplest are the jug-type filters, using loose, activated charcoal (usually produced from coconut husks) but carbon filtration can be rather elaborate using loose, activated block filters and/or block filters. The simplest types do a great job reducing chlorine concentration, gases, odours and taste, but do very little to protect against other contaminants. Some of the more comprehensive (read expensive) types such as large carbon block filters will also reduce the concentration of some pesticides, other organic compounds and heavy metals. Carbon filters, especially the small, loose carbon type, should be changed at regular intervals as they will build up potentially hazardous levels of bacteria and at saturation can start to unload toxins back into the 'filtered' water. Silver or ultra-violet bactericidal units are sometimes attached between plumbed-in carbon filters and the faucet in order to control bacteria that

can readily develop. Again, many people don't use simple, jug-type carbon filters for their cooking water or to fill up their kettle.

3. **Ceramic filters**. These are made of clay, volcanic sand or magnetite stone. They are particularly good at removing heavy metals, other inorganic compounds (including nitrates and fluoride) and bacteria and cysts. The weakness of ceramic filters is the poor removal of organic compounds like pesticides, dioxins and oestrogens. They have the benefit of being long-lasting and can be cleaned by the user. Water flow rates are normally slow so that people tend to use ceramic filters mainly just for drinking purposes.
4. **Distilled water.** These are some of the most expensive systems for home installation and basically rely on the process of collecting the steam from boiling water. Distillers make the purest water. Some argue that such pure water can actually leach minerals from the body but pure water cannot attract organically-bound minerals out of our bones or bodies in the manner claimed. Evidence for the fact that pure water does not leach minerals out of the body comes from the many tens of thousands of kidney patients using distilled water in dialysis machines who show no loss of mineral content in their bodies. One of the biggest drawbacks with distillation systems is their high purchase price.
5. **Reverse osmosis-based filtration systems**. In many ways, state-of-the-art plumbed-in reverse osmosis systems give you the best of carbon technology combined with the benefits of reverse osmosis filtration. Reverse osmosis (RO) is a complicated process which uses a membrane under pressure to separate relatively pure water (or other solvent) from a less pure solution. When two aqueous solutions of different concentrations are separated by a semi-permeable membrane, water passes through the membrane in the direction of the more concentrated solution as a result of osmotic pressure. If enough counter pressure is applied to the concentrated solution to overcome the osmotic pressure, the flow of water will be reversed. RO membranes typically have pore sizes of 0.0005 microns so water is generally

produced slowly and stored in a tank. Once lime added to tap water has been removed, the water tends to be slightly acidic, but for the reasons given for distilled water this does not appear to be problematic in practice. Some companies are able to attach 'mineralisers' to their systems so that minerals can be added back to the water, so stabilising the pH. Obviously we should recognise that organic forms of minerals as found in foods are much more easily absorbed by the body than elemental forms. Combined carbon/RO systems produce water that is of a similar composition to rainwater. They are very efficient at removing or very substantially reducing the concentration of the full spectrum of organic and inorganic contaminants, pathogens and radio-active compounds. The carbon filters tend to need annual replacement, while the RO membranes can generally be used for two to four years before replacement is required.

APPENDIX II

GM foods – Weapons of Mass Destruction?

(Reproduced from **icon** August 2003)

Move over, Darwin

Organic food, much prized by Cancer Therapists from Issels to Gerson, or Plaskett to Contreras, is under threat. This time from a unique form of pollution, a form that is believed to have polluted 11 per cent of the total acreage in the USA already, and has some scientists estimating that in 10 years there could simply be no true organic food left in the USA at all.

This pollution is a genetic variant that a million years of evolution has failed to spawn. If Darwinian theory is to be believed, we are what we are today solely because of millions of genetic changes, some enabling us to grow stronger, many simply generating weakness in organisms that fell by the way-side.

Well all that is changing. Now scientists can make a genetic modification in the DNA of crops, one that may have happened a zillion times before; or is it something that has never happened in this format before? Either way, biotech companies believe genetically modified crops will benefit us all in the long run. But are they right or is this just the pursuit of profits by bullyboys in large offices?

Worse, as many people fear, are we not simply letting loose the equivalent of a computer virus into our green and pleasant land? A virus that simply cannot be stopped once it is introduced. We have already had the reports that cloned animals seem to be weaker than normally produced equivalents. Scientists who experiment can never say anything with certainty. After all, that is the essence of experimentation. What if the same is true for Genetically Modified crops? An experiment waiting to go horribly wrong? Not in the first five years but during the lives of our children, or during the lives of our children's children? Armageddon, irreversibly programmed into the food chain?

Now, the biotech scientists are ready, I'm sure, to label me a scaremonger. One of them was quoted in the Press in October 2003 as saying that the modified DNA would be broken down into its constituent parts long before it could cross the intestine wall and into your blood system. Frankly, that argument is rubbish. It's simply not true; even if we all had perfect guts, which we haven't, without any leaks. If a microbe or a fungus can cross the gut wall, what hope a much smaller piece of DNA?

And then what happens? Can someone reassure me that there is absolutely no chance of a combination with any of my DNA in any one cell of my body? For what is cancer if it is not genetic modification?

The potential for chaos is clear. If Messrs Bush and Blair are looking for weapons of mass destruction, they could do well to start on the plains of the mid-west of America.

It's decision time

Notwithstanding the possibility that it could be too late already, in autumn 2003 there will be a Government decision whether or not to allow the commercial growing of GM crops in Britain. Sadly, yet again our Government demonstrates its abilities to focus on the wrong issues.

Lord Sainsbury – the man who feels nobility (in the form of Prince Charles but, of course, not himself) should keep out of political issues – is lobbying hard for GM food in Britain. But then he is The Science Minister, he should know all about the facts on GM foods.

The argument for GM?

The 'pro lobby' has three main claims: third world poverty decreases, productivity increases, and herbicide and pesticide decreases. Except that the third world debt is more likely to rise with GM foods as crop growers are not allowed to collect seed and thus have to buy new seed every year from the manufacturers. And to date there is no confirmed research that productivity rises with GM food while, anyway, the WHO already says that worldwide we produce more food than we need.

Finally, so far, there is absolutely no scientific evidence that less pesticides and herbicides will be needed. And anyway, the original idea was that since the chemicals killed some of the crops as well as the weeds and pests, the gene mutation would be incorporated to allow the same spraying to continue but with less food loss! No one originally said anything about using less chemicals.

So far, so bad. Lord Sainsbury – you are off to a pretty poor start!

The 'let's wait five years for test results' strategy

Here the main rationale seems to be a desire to see to what degree growing GM crops damages the environment. If this had been a 'proper' scientific test – the sort that western governments expect from top quality clinical drug trials, (and let's be honest – how much faith do you really have in those? It would be irresponsible of me to mention Thalidomide) there would have been 'pre-research' evidence, monitoring during the tests and a 'control'. After all Genetically Modified foods could well have a toxic, drug like effect on our bodies maybe not immediate but over time – no one has scientific evidence to counter that theory. So in the case of GM foods, the equivalent to clinical trials might have been to take a couple of fields in a distant part of Norfolk or Cornwall and measure various factors – like wildlife decline, or spread of pollen – at distances of 100 yards, 500 yards, 1 km etc against life in a normal equivalent and distant control region. That's a proper scientific study.

Instead we have a patchwork of possible pollution throughout the country. Judges who have little knowledge of science, let alone wind effects or the abilities of birds and other wildlife to spread pollen, seem to have made random decisions to allow GM foods 60 yards (or was it feet?), from a field growing organic food.

This is not science. This is nonsense. Michael Meacher did make a very strong case against all this – sadly this is his area of influence no more.

So what will we have measured, Lord Sainsbury? Did we do a stock check on wild birds before the tests? Will we study the pollen pollution at various distances afterwards? Did we attempt to localise the tests to that if the worst happens and there is widespread pollution, we still may have some natural organic crops left at the end of the five years? In the USA, 11 per cent of organic farmers have experienced pollution to date.

Fortunately, Friends of the Earth have been looking into this for us. At a test site on Humberside, pollen has been found over a mile away. In research actually funded by FoE pollen was found in a beehive three miles from a test field.

Already there are fears of superweeds because a number of weeds are actually closely related to some of the commercial crops, making cross pollination that much more likely. Wild Turnip, Wild Cabbage, Wild Radish, Hoary and Brown Mustard are all weeds but there is already proven cross pollination by oilseed rape. And what do we intend to grow commercially? Genetically modified oilseed rape.

In the UK this weapon of mass destruction could potentially create superweeds covering most of England and Wales. Why, oh why, are we even thinking of allowing it?

But what about my health?

While we are busy measuring (or not) the health of our crops and our weeds, what about measuring the effects on my health? The BMA has already warned that there is not enough evidence to say GM foods are safe.

Do you realise that to date there has been no large scale scientific studies at all on the effects of actually eating the GM crops!? Of course there's a lot of scientific pooh-poohing along the lines of 'well even if the DNA has been modified, you just break it down in the digestive process so it cannot harm you'. Twaddle. Who says? Our bodies have evolved, along with their DNA, to be in balance with our environments over the last few hundred thousand years. One of our biggest threats – and the reason why cancer seems to be taking such a hold in the modern world – is that our environment has changed so dramatically over the last 150 years that our evolution cannot react fast enough! So, pray tell me, how is a five-year study supposed to tell us what the **long-term effects** on my (and my children's) genetic code are likely to be?

Mao Tse Tung was asked by a French diplomat, what he

thought about the French revolution. He answered that, 'it was too early to tell!' It's a shame he is not our Science Minister.

Where crops are concerned our standard health measurements involve discussions on vitamins and minerals. An area completely overlooked is the life energy system. As soon as people talk body energy or auras to most medical people, eyebrows get raised and medical authorities become quite dismissive. 'Eastern mumbo-jumbo' is about the best response you get. But the fact is that natural organic food has large energy fields, non-organic foods have smaller ones, and five day old non-organic food (the sort you get in supermarkets) the least. Which medical authority can disprove my theory that when I eat a vegetable I gain its vitamins, minerals and natural energy? Maybe the energy consumed is even more important to my health than the vitamins and minerals.

Which scientific authority will tell me if GM food has the same energy level as organic food? If it doesn't need pesticides then you would have thought this might be a benefit. But no one is looking in this direction. I have this terrible feeling that in 50 years time, when the true importance of body energy, auras and magnetic fields to our everyday health is fully known and appreciated, our grand children will look back on current times in horror.

From America are coming the first reports of one potential problem. Some GM crops are designed to kill bugs. All bugs. So what happens to the good bugs in our stomach? Already there are emerging stories that the good guys in our stomachs can be destroyed by the GM foods.

As we saw in June's **icon**, if you destroy the friendly flora, you open a Pandora's box of problems. Fungi and microbes are free to multiply; they devour vitamins ordinarily destined to nourish you, produce toxins (even carcinogenic ones) and a waste alcohol on which cancer cells thrive.

From Canada, there is also a small scale research study on 280 male chickens. Half were fed with T25 (a Chardon GM LL maize from Aventis/Bayer) and over a 42 day test period the death rate in the GM sample was twice that in the control sample. In a bizarre twist, this research study was actually submitted by the manufacturers as evidence for the GM maize's safety! Worse, the

UK Advisory Committee on Releases to the Environment (ACRE) actually approved it!!

From Argentina, where GM crops have been present for a number of years, comes a report that in the first two years of planting, herbicide levels were only 5–10 per cent of previous levels. However, as the superweeds have grown, the Argentinians now use even more herbicides than they did before GM foods, thus defeating the whole object.

So please Mr Blair, let us not make a decision without real studies and real beefy scientific evidence, not merely on the crops but, more importantly, on the humans that eat them (who coincidentally are voters). My children's health is more important than the profits of a few US companies.

Oh, and let's leave the decision until a sensible length of study has elapsed. For example, about 20,000 years.

APPENDIX III

Liver Cleanse / Gallstone Flush

Ingredients:

$^1/_2$ cup extra virgin olive oil
1 very big grapefruit (providing $^3/_4$ cup of juice)
4 tablespoons of Epsom Salts
3 cups of water
Ornithine tablets.

Preparation:

Set aside 3 days.

Day 1:

Eat a no-fat breakfast and lunch.
Eat and drink nothing after 2.00 pm.
Mix the Epsom Salts in the water (easier if water is warm), then cool.

6.00 pm	Drink a quarter of this liquid.
8.00 pm	Drink a further quarter of the liquid
10.00 pm	Mix the olive oil and pulp-free grapefruit juice and shake vigorously. Drink the liquid through a straw before 10.15 pm. Take four Ornithine tablets to help you sleep. Retire immediately and massage your stomach. Focus your mind on your liver and imagine the toxins leaving it, along with the stones. Sleep.

Day 2:

Upon waking and not before 7.00 am take the third quarter of the Epsom salts mix. Two hours later take the last quarter.

Expect diarrhoea for two days; don't eat before lunch time on day two and keep food to salads and fruit, plus baked potatoes for days two and three.

You may need to repeat this treatment after a few weeks. 2000–3000 small stones may be passed.

Please note – This recipe is derived from William Kelley's cancer treatment. It has thousands of testimonials, none report pain, only success; but nobody at **icon** has any first hand experience of it. And although a number of our readers have now tried the 'treatment and been happy with the results, we are merely **told** it works!

APPENDIX IV

Acid Residue Products – a fuller list

FRUITS
- Bananas
- Grapefruit
- Oranges
- Plums
- Prunes

VEGETABLES
- Asparagus tips
- Brussel sprouts
- Chick peas
- Dried beans
- Lentils
- Peanuts
- Rhubarb
- Tomatoes

ALL DAIRY

ALL FLESH FOODS
- Meats, fish, shellfish, scallops, crab,
- All processed and salted meats, smoked fish

CEREALS AND NUTS
- All packet nuts, crisps and snacks
- All refined flour including noodles, spaghetti, buckwheat
- Barley
- Cornflakes and most processed breakfast cereals
- Doughnuts
- Dumplings
- Macaroni
- Oatmeal
- Pies, pastries and bread
- Refined rice

OTHER
- All alcohol
- Chocolate, cocoa
- Coffee, tea
- Fizzy drinks
- Eggs
- Lack of sleep
- Negative emotions
- Preservatives, jams, etc.
- Products in vinegar
- Salt and condiments
- Sauces
- Stress
- Sugar
- Sweets
- Tobacco
- Vinegar

Alkaline Residue Products - a fuller list

FRESH FRUITS

- Apple
- Apricot
- Avocado
- Blackberries
- Blackcurrants
- Cherries
- Cranberries
- Currants, raisins
- Dates
- Figs
- Grapes
- Lemons
- Lychees
- Mangoes
- Melon
- Olives
- Papaya
- Peach
- Pear
- Raspberries
- Redcurrants

OTHER

- Alfalfa
- Agar-Agar
- Fresh cracked nuts
- Fresh ginger
- Fresh juices (own preparation)
- Herb teas, green tea
- Honey
- Millet
- Noni juice
- Olive oil, corn oil
- Seeds
- Soya products

VEGETABLES

- Aubergines
- Beetroot
- Broccoli
- Cabbage
- Carrots, parsnips
- Cauliflower
- Celery
- Chard
- Chicory
- Chives
- Cucumber
- Dandelion
- Dill
- Endive
- Fresh green beans
- Garlic
- Kale
- Kelp
- Lettuce
- Mushrooms
- Parsnips
- Peppers
- Potatoes
- Radishes
- Sorrel
- Soya beans
- Spinach
- Squash
- Swede
- Turnips
- Watercress

REFERENCES

1. Simone, C.B. (1992) *Cancer and Nutrition.* Avery Publishing: New York.
2. Beazley, *The Betrayal of Health.*
3. Page, Harris, Epstein, *Drinking Water in Louisiana.*
4. Carlo, Mettlin, *Cancer Incidence and Trihalomethane Concentrations in Public Water Systems.*
5. Campbell, A. (2002) 'The potential role of aluminium in Alzheimer's disease'. *Nephrology Dialysis Transplantation 17: 17, 20.*
6. Varner, J.A., Jensen, K.F., Horvath, W., Isaacson, R.L. (1998) 'Chronic administration of aluminium fluoride or sodium fluoride to rats in drinking water; alterations in neuronal and cerebrovascular integrity'. *Brain Research, 784: 284–298.*

To order more copies of this book

Tel: 44(0)1280 815166
Fax: 44(0)1280 824655
Email: enquiries@iconmag.co.uk

OESTROGEN

THE KILLER IN OUR MIDST

by

Chris Woollams

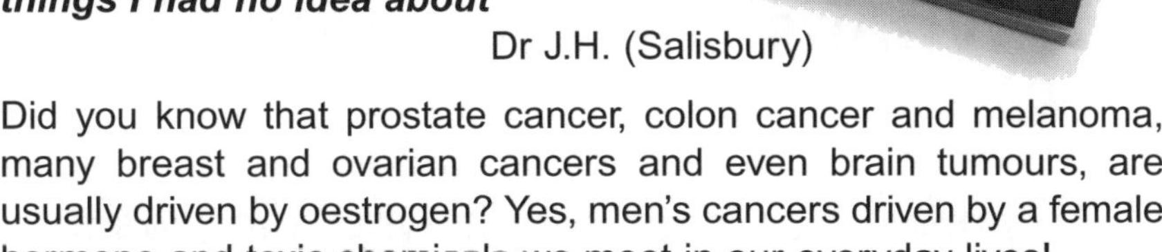

"This book is amazing – it told me things I had no idea about"

Dr J.H. (Salisbury)

Did you know that prostate cancer, colon cancer and melanoma, many breast and ovarian cancers and even brain tumours, are usually driven by oestrogen? Yes, men's cancers driven by a female hormone and toxic chemicals we meet in our everyday lives!

Some specialists believe 90 per cent of solid cancers are hormonally driven and 90 per cent of these we prove are driven by oestrogen. And this is true for both men and women.

Chris says: *"This book is a very important book for anyone with a solid tumour. It is meant to be very easy and quick to read, but to clearly cover the facts and suggest what action you might take to amplify your orthodox treatment. Things most doctors simply do not tell you. It will also save me a lot of time. Hormonally driven cancer is so common I have often had the same conversation five times in just a few hours!"*

Oestrogen: The Killer in Our Midst is a self-help book for all those wishing to beat or avoid hormonally responsive cancer.

"It's easy to read and with a checklist of action points. It pulls all the information together in a usable way."

E.T. (Hertfordshire)

"I think it's invaluable for anyone, male or female. It covers everything from cutting oestrogen excesses out of your life to the use of natural progesterone. I didn't realise that there is so much you can do."

P. F. (Limerick, Eire)

Tel: 44(0)1280 815166

Fax: 44(0)1280 824655

E-mail: enquiries@iconmag.co.uk

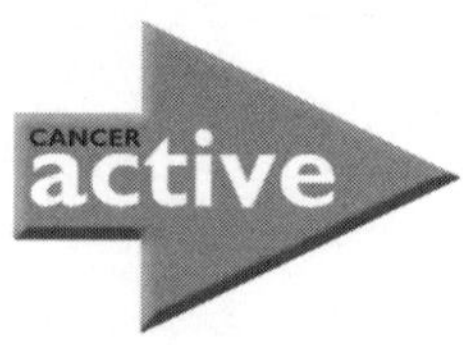

CANCERactive is a new charity with three important points of difference.

- First, it brings you the WHOLE TRUTH ON CANCER TREATMENTS: all the up-to-date facts about every researched therapy that might be of help to you. From surgery to supplements; from radiotherapy to exercise; from chemotherapy to photodynamic therapy. We don't show bias, we just lay out the facts so you can choose.
- Second, it is dedicated to helping people build an INTEGRATED treatment programme, to maximise their chances of survival. Books, a magazine (**icon**) and an easy-to-follow website are all packed with information and our own research is planned.
- Third, it aims to take the PREVENTION message where it matters, into schools and to parents.

BECOME AN ACTIVIST – JOIN THE FORCE

For just 50 pence per week you can join the FORCE, and receive **icon** posted to your home, a monthly e-newsletter, discounts on health products and a whole lot more.

"Everything you need to know to help you beat cancer."

Now no one need die of ignorance

Tel: 44(0)1280 815166
Fax: 44(0)1280 824655
E-mail: enquiries@iconmag.co.uk

Bill Farlow's

RVing From A to Z

Here at last, by public demand

Veteran RV writer Bill Farlow, in response to appeals from his readers, has finally authored a book containing no-nonsense advice on how to get the most fun and best performance out of RVs, tow vehicles and dozens of key accessories that are indispensable to the RV lifestyle.

A full-time RVer, Farlow has built almost a cult following among the kindred souls who read publications such as *Trailer Life, Camp-Orama, Trails-A-Way, Southern RV, Coast to Coast, Camperways* and others.

Beginning with the chapter "50 Things Your Dealer Never Told You," Farlow doesn't hesitate to tell it as he sees it. Here are a sampling of the subjects covered by this popular author:

- **Air conditioners**
- **Selecting batteries**
- **Engine heat**
- **Overdrive/underdrive**
- **Hoses, cords, adapters**
- **Engine tuning**
- **Selecting tires**
- **Upper cylinder lubricants**
- **Weights and GVWRs**
- **Attic fans**
- **Brake care**
- **Gear ratios**
- **Hitches**
- **Manuals**
- **Spark plugs**
- **Turbochargers**
- **Vapor lock**
- **Winterizing**

Bill Farlow's

RVing From A to Z

BY BILL FARLOW

Edited by Don Wright

First printing 1991
Second printing 1993
Printed in the United States of America

Bill Farlow's RVING FROM A TO Z

ISBN 0-937877-07-7

Cottage Publications, Inc.
24396 Pleasant View Dr., Elkhart, IN 46517 (219/875-8618)